Continuity and Crisis in the NHS

The Politics of Design and Innovation in Health Care

*Edited by Ray Loveridge
and Ken Starkey*

Open University Press
Buckingham ● *Philadelphia*

Open University Press
Celtic Court
22 Ballmoor
Buckingham
MK18 1XW

and

1900 Frost Road, Suite 101
Bristol, PA 19007, USA

First Published 1992

A catalogue record of this book is available from the British Library

Library of Congress Cataloging-in-Publication Data

Continuity and crisis in the NHS: the politics of design and
    innovation in health care/edited by Ray Loveridge and Ken Starkey.
        p.   cm.
    Includes bibliographical references and index.
    ISBN 0–335–15599–5 (paper) – ISBN 0–335–15620–7 (cased)
    1. National Health Service (Great Britain)   I. Loveridge, Ray.
II. Starkey, Ken, 1948–   .
    [DNLM: 1. Delivery of Health Care – organization & administration –
Great Britain.   2. Delivery of Health Care – trends – Great Britain.
3. State Medicine – organization & administration – Great Britain.
4. State Medicine – trends – Great Britain.   W 275 FA1 C76]
RA395.G6C645   1992
362.1'0941 – dc20
DNLM/DLC
for Library of Congress   91–32169
                                                                         CIP

E·S·R·C
ECONOMIC
& SOCIAL
RESEARCH
COUNCIL

Typeset by Graphicraft Typesetters Ltd, Hong Kong
Printed in Great Britain by Biddles Ltd, Guildford and King's Lynn

Dedicated to the innovative life of Sheri Ahmad

Contents

List of Contributors

Sheri Ahmad (deceased), Formerly Consultant in Accident and Emergency Medicine, Dudley District Health Authority.

Alison Blenkinsopp, Lecturer in Community Pharmacy, University of Bradford.

Peter Bryden, General Practitioner of Medicine, Hastings District Health Authority.

Rod Coombs, Senior Lecturer and Director of CROMTEC, University of Manchester, Institute of Science and Technology.

David Cooper, Professor of Accountancy, University of Manchester, Institute of Science and Technology.

David Cox, Senior Lecturer, Birmingham Business School, Birmingham Polytechnic.

Peter G. Davey, Senior Lecturer in Pharmacology and Infectious Diseases, Department of Clinical Pharmacology, Ninewells Hospital, University of Dundee.

Michael Dent, Senior Lecturer in Sociology, Staffordshire Polytechnic.

Ruth Green, Lecturer in Sociology, Staffordshire Polytechnic.

Sheila Greenfield, Senior Lecturer, The Medical School, University of Birmingham.

Margaret Grieco, Research Fellow, Transport Studies Unit, University of Oxford.

Ray Loveridge, Professor and Head of Strategic Management and Policy Studies, Aston Business School.

Mo H. Malek, Lecturer in Management, University of St. Andrews.

William Scott, Chief Administrator, Pharmaceutical Office, Tayside Health Board, Dundee.

Sudi Sharifi, Lecturer in Management and Organizational Behaviour, University of Birmingham.

Brian Shaw, Reader in Management, Oxford Polytechnic.

Judy Smith, Lecturer in Sociology, Staffordshire Polytechnic.

Ken Starkey, Reader in Organizational Analysis, University of Nottingham.

Gary Vann-Wye, Research Associate, Aston Business School.

Foreword

This book sets out to examine innovation in the UK National Health Service (NHS). It represents a collection of work by academics, clinicians and others who have worked in the NHS and been involved at the grassroots level in trying to implement change in the service. The book examines key areas of the NHS change agenda: management systems, the nature of professionalism, strategic management, occupational and organizational change, new initiatives in health care provision and the impact of new technology, including the new information technologies. This examination is set in the context of a critical analysis of the overall innovation process in health care. The emphasis is on the negotiation of power within the change process. It is hoped that these illustrations will provide a basis for an intelligent unravelling of the likely results of the Government's action – both that initiated by the Thatcher Administration between 1979 and 1990 and that of its successors. The application of general management principles to the NHS during the 1980s represents a fundamental challenge to traditional modes of health service delivery (Strong and Robinson, 1990). Whatever the political regime of the future the expanded role of a professional managerial cadre in health care has come to stay even if its actual form and focus differ over time. Despite or perhaps because of this the lessons contained in this volume are likely to need to be learnt and relearnt over coming decades.

The book has its origins in the work of the Economic and Social Research Council's Work Organization Research Centre at Aston Business School during the 1980s. The Centre undertook a series of longitudinal studies of design and innovation in a variety of industries in both the private and public sectors (see, for example, Clark and Starkey, 1988;

Starkey and McKinlay, 1988; Child and Loveridge, 1990; Loveridge and Pitt, 1990). Several of the authors represented in this collection worked in or were affiliated to the Work Organization Research Centre. Others are colleagues with whom the Centre collaborated in its work within various Regions of the NHS. The book, therefore, represents a view from the geographical centre of the UK but it also encompasses the country's extremities!

Various drafts of the book have been processed, in every sense of the word, by Caroline Etchells, and, more latterly, by Julie Ellen. The authors owe them a considerable debt for this final version. Before the book could be published, the author of one of its most vivid accounts of innovation, Sheri Ahmad, a consultant from the Dudley District General Hospital, suffered a fatal heart attack. His chapter reminds us of the loss suffered by the NHS in the passing of this enormously talented and charming person.

Plan of the book

The dynamics of change are explored from two perspectives. The first perspective focusses on attempted innovation in NHS management practices. It analyses the issues of managerialism and professionalism as they developed as principles of NHS administration and their impact on occupational, organizational and strategic change in the NHS during the 1980s. The second perspective focusses on innovations in technology. Included are several studies of the neglected area of hospital planning and design.

In Chapter 1, Loveridge and Starkey present a general introduction of the twin themes of innovation in management practice and innovation in technology, including a critical examination of the possible implications of the 1989 White Paper, *Working for Patients*. Chapter 2 by Cox addresses the conflict in values contained within the introduction of the new managerialism in the NHS. He suggests that the notion of a commodified form of service delivery which forms the basis of the discourse of the new managerialism detracts from a shared moral commitment to client welfare that has, previously, provided cohesion, perhaps the only cohesion, across the apparently disparate groups making up the NHS. He contrasts the new image of the client as 'consumer' that marks the Thatcherite reforms with the earlier ideal of 'citizenship'.

In Chapter 3, Malek *et al.* examine patterns of doctors' prescribing behaviour and attempts to change these in one health authority. They suggest that a great deal of medical power derives from the doctor's gatekeeper position in the manufacturing chains that supply goods and services to the point of care delivery. The doctor's role as agent for the consumer enables the medical profession to affect the purchasing policies of the NHS in its dealings with manufacturers and in particular with the pharmaceutical industry. Instead of the application of clear evaluative routines based on scientific testing to prescribing behaviours the authors discover in clinical practice a wide variety of prescribing standards and a deep involvement of doctors in the high pressure sales campaigns run by producers. They look to the development of the professional role of community pharmacists as offering a more rigorous filtering process in the drug adoption process and a superior rationality to decisions in this crucial area of NHS expenditure. In doing so they raise a crucial theme for the remainder of the book – the issue of the locus of control concerning key operational and expenditure decisions.

The theme of control is further developed in the next four chapters which focus on current changes in the work and market situation of NHS professionals. In Chapter 4, Starkey finds the desire of consultants and general practitioners (GPs) for more time-specific contracts to be part of a trend towards the commodification of their time. He argues that this can only lead to their eventual subordination to managerialism and, thus, threatens their autonomy in respect to other aspects of their task situation.

Bryden, a practising GP, suggests a different interpretation of changes currently taking place in GP contracts. He argues in Chapter 5 that the new contract for GPs, together with the Government's proposals for budget-holding general practices, will enable the re-birth of an early ideal of the founders of the NHS, the community clinic. He further argues that increasingly effective professional administration over the primary care team at the point of delivery will free the GP to practise medicine as never before. New information technology will facilitate the rationalization of service delivery with the GP as the agent of this process. Bryden, therefore, sees a different outcome than the one suggested by Starkey of a possible disempowerment of medical professionals under the gaze of the new managerial elite. But both authors see the power of the medical professional as a crucial issue in the innovation process. For Bryden's vision to become reality, it is the balance of power between doctors that must change as the consultant accommodates to the enhanced management role of the GP.

The next two chapters probe the reality behind Bryden's aspirations for community care but from the perspectives of groups other than doctors. Greenfield, in Chapter 6, investigates the extent to which nurse practitioners are capable of assuming many of the patient screening and routine treatment duties in general practices. Perhaps inevitably in the UK context, she is forced to the conclusion that the responsibilities of nurses in general practice already outrun the availability of training facilities or the acknowledgement of the formal institutions. As in several other areas of nursing within the NHS this situation leaves the incumbents of such extended roles in a dangerously exposed situation relative to current law. But, with an increasing recognition of an expanded role for the nurse, the potential for economies in service provision, particularly in expensive doctor time, becomes a more realistic possibility.

In Chapter 7, Blenkinsopp surveys the latest stage in a 200-year-old dispute between physicians and pharmacists triggered by the Nuffield

Inquiry and subsequent White Paper of 1987. These documents proposed an extended role for pharmacists which included access to patients in the community, a physician's monopoly since the mid-19th century (Parry and Parry, 1976). Again, the issue of a possible re-think of the role of the various occupational groups in the provision of primary care becomes of increasing importance. Blenkinsopp's chapter provides hope for pharmacists in the more perfect market that could be created by information technology. The variety of materials used in dispensing and the formulated nature of the task has created a context for rapid computerization. Pharmacists have also become the UK pioneers of the SMART card which enables the client to possess their own portable record of treatments. This form of direct client access to the system runs counter to current medical philosophy in which a doctor has always to act as the consumer's agent in the selection of the appropriate diagnosis and treatment of ailments.

In Chapter 8 the focus of the book shifts to its second major theme: the management of technological change. This is first addressed by Shaw in his analysis of the unique role played by clinicians in the invention, design, testing and implementation of new equipment in health care delivery. This research reaffirms the remarkable control exercised by physicians over the market for manufactured supplies which was referred to in Chapter 3.

In Chapter 9, Coombs and Cooper pursue the issue of financial control. They see recent reforms in the NHS being diffused through the media of financial software packages and accounting conventions. Taking as their starting point the recommendation of the Griffiths Report that doctors should be the 'natural managers' of the service, the devolution of resource management to consultants and GPs is seen as broadening during the 1990s. While apparently offering greater financial autonomy they argue that this process will also co-opt doctors into a process designed to monitor their own activities from the centre. The authors point to the likely obstacles to the process as its political nature is increasingly contested.

The divergent manner in which four District Health Authorities responded to a strategic initiative in information technology (IT) is described by Dent *et al.* in Chapter 10. The existence of a management capability to absorb the changes in both practice and knowledge differed across the different authorities. There were also different systems of control and coordination in operation in the four locations, in spite of the apparently standardized formal structures promulgated throughout the service. Bureaucratic rationality, therefore, seems to be locally, as opposed to nationally, specific. In Chapter 11 the late Sheri Ahmad, who was a practising consultant, sets out in a very presonal way the frustrations he experienced in designing and implementing one of the first computerized patient information systems to be installed in an Accident and Emergency Department in the UK. Medical power in practice had to come to terms with the problems of bureaucracy and administrative incompetence.

Chapter 12 extends our consideration of technological change to the history and current implementation of changes in the design of hospitals.

Vann-Wye traces the development of competing technologies of care from the last century to the present day in order to explain the current success of what he describes as individualistic-curative methodologies over communal-preventative. He outlines the successive unsuccessful attempts to standardize and to industrialize, thus to rationalize, hospital design on a national basis since the 1950s.

In Chapter 13 Sharifi pursues the same theme of hospital design. She considers the extent to which the decision makers in the design of a new District General Hospital were influenced by a complex of cultural norms as well as by national guidelines in a manner that precluded 'rational' consideration of all objectively available options. The politicality of the decision-making process is a key element of Sharifi's analysis. In Chapter 14, Grieco extends the analysis of political constraints on innovation and the limits to the rational uptake of new treatment design. She observes the manner in which the concept of the central treatment area introduced in standardized hospital design packages promulgated by the former DHSS in the 1970s became utilized in two entirely different modes of treatment delivery in separate hospitals built to these standards. She concludes that the local structures of custom and practice that emerged reflect the cultural predispositions of the pioneers, the local champions of central treatment at each of the sites, rather than national design standards.

Finally, in Chapter 15 Loveridge argues that the continuation of technological innovation in health care delivery will inevitably involve the greater participation of professional care-providers in its management. The knowledge base used in professional socialization is likely to extend to the techniques of management as a means of defending a traditional area of professional authority. Without such involvement it is unlikely that the systemic behavioural change sought for at the point of delivery will take place.

References

Child, J. and Loveridge, R. (1990) *Information Technology in European Services*. Oxford: Basil Blackwell.

Clark, P. and Starkey, K. (1988) *Organization Transitions and Innovation-Design*. London: Pinter Publishers.

Loveridge, R. and Pitt, M. (eds) (1990) *The Strategic Management of Technological Innovation*. Chichester: John Wiley.

Parry, N. and Parry, J. (1976) *The Rise of the Medical Profession*. London: Croom Helm.

Starkey, K. and McKinlay, A. (1988) *Organizational Innovation*. Aldershot, Gower.

Strong, P. and Robinson, J. (1990) *The NHS Under New Management*. Milton Keynes: Open University Press.

1 | Introduction: Innovation and Interest in the Organization of Health Care Delivery

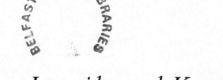

Ray Loveridge and Ken Starkey

The changes envisaged in the management of health care delivery set out in the National Health Service and Community Care Act (1990) were indubitably the most radical since Aneurin Bevan presided over the birth of a national system for the whole of the UK in 1948. The underlying purpose of these changes – that of introducing competition between carers in order to promote greater economy and managerial efficiency – has been seen by many critics as undermining the citizen's right of access to professionally guided treatment. Others such as Powell (1966) have long argued for the setting of constraints on the mounting cost of health care through the adoption of overt bases for rationing. The finally adopted strategy, that of uncoupling hierarchical linkages between primary and secondary care, evidently owed much to the ideas of another, American, academic analyst. The suggestions put forward by Professor Enthoven in 1985 for the creation of an internal market between 'providers' of a service and 'purchasers' resonated with the prevailing spirit of economic liberalism rather better than those of previous proposals for bureaucratic constraints on care deliverers.

Both sets of analysts have recognized that in the UK National Health Service (NHS) they were confronted with an institutional environment grounded in organized politics and an on-going internal struggle for the control of scarce resources. As a result, while there was a consensus that the NHS was faced with a crisis that combined a growing lack of resources with incipient lack of credibility, there was little agreement within the NHS about how its managers should respond to this crisis. The absence of an accepted agenda for change in the NHS over much of its life had resulted in an appearance of operational inertia in its management.

This is, in fact, how many observers have characterized the strategic performance of the NHS over the past 40 and more years of its existence. In practice, for at least half of that time, new directions have been set by government and the Department of Health with some regularity but little operational effect. Like health administration in most parts of the world the day-to-day management of its operations has displayed a continuity, and even conservatism, that has contrasted with the apparent pace of social and economic change. Moreover, the apparent lack of ability to discover administrative solutions for its multiplying problems has increasingly contrasted with the speed of innovation in the diagnosis and treatment of physical diseases within the NHS. It is this disjunction that recurs throughout this volume. The resource providers would obviously wish to retain the creativity and inventiveness of medical care-providers whilst structuring these activities in a manner that will allow for the greater standardization and monitoring of performance. It is by no means clear that the latter goals can be achieved without seriously impeding the operational autonomy seen by the creative provider of care to be essential to his or her professional performance.

The problem outlined above is not unknown to students of organizational management. A large part of the literature that still forms the core of teaching across the disciplines making up operational management is focussed on the formal measurement of efficiency and economy. Social scientists, by contrast, have emphasized the political aspects of organization behaviour that have important consequences for effectiveness and innovation. Organizations find it difficult to change. The *status quo* tends to be sustained by powerful sub-groups who legitimate the prevailing value and meaning systems (Miles, 1980). Indeed the preoccupation of these sub-groups with the preservation of their social and market territories may be such that, in spite of enormous internal activity, the social system of which they are part remains static. Most of the case studies in this volume explore just such conditions. They are intended to provide insights into the 'evolutionary context', according to Kimberley (1982, p. 641):

> those patterns of development which antedate any particular organisation/innovation interaction [and] influence the atmosphere in which that interaction unfolds

thus affecting the behaviour of key actors and the ultimate fate of the innovation. The effect of tradition and its stifling effects on organizational evolution has been characterized in terms of managerial recipes (Grinyer and Spender, 1979). Managers are socialized into particular organizational patterns of action and their behaviour becomes routinized as they believe that what they have learnt is time- and context-free, a 'one best way' of coping with problems facing their organization. The present is constantly interpreted and fitted into perceptions governed by recipes constructed on the basis of past experience.

To the extent that the environment in which an organization exists and with which it interacts is stable and predictable, the management of change can afford to be incremental. Marginal improvements to tried and tested ways of performing the organization's work will suffice. But when the organization's environment changes radically, becoming more complex and less predictable, recipes are soon outmoded and become a liability rather than an assurance of organizational effectiveness and survival. In this chapter, and in those that follow, the social roots of cultural continuity in the NHS are traced by the authors in an effort to understand the obstacles to present radical changes. Without this qualitative understanding of present relationships it seems impossible either to measure the efficacy of current innovations in formal procedures or to anticipate their outcomes.

New directions

Strategic direction for the administration of the NHS in the UK has always been set by the Secretary of State for Health who has been a member of the Cabinet and responsible to Parliament since the inception of the NHS in 1948. Since 1988 its planning and articulation has been the responsibility of the Chief Executive and Board working through the Department of Health (DoH) (formerly the Department of Health and Social Security (DHSS)). Below national level, eleven Regional Health Authorities (RHAs) have responsibility for much of strategic implementation, particularly as it applies to capital investment. Within each region services are provided through a number of channels, the most significant of which are those of the District Health Authority's (DHA) provisions of hospital or secondary services and those of the Family Health Service Authorities (FHSA, formerly known as the Family Practitioners Committees) who, with local government, provide community or primary care. Of the large proportion of gross domestic product (about 9 per cent) spent on health care by the state, the bulk (about 80 per cent) is channelled into hospital-based treatments.

The broad effect of the National Health Service and Community Care Act (1990) has been to create a class of consumers' agents in the FHSAs who will, acting through GPs, buy the services provided by the DHA hospitals. These two sets of authorities will also be responsible for monitoring and auditing the standards of service offered on behalf of the RHAs and DoH.

A fairly crucial trigger to activating these structural reforms envisaged in the 1990 Act was contained in the right accorded both to GPs and to hospitals to opt for becoming independent agents for the purposes of setting prices for their services, in the case of hospitals, and for shopping around for value in referring patients to hospitals by GPs. This trigger could only be activated if sufficient numbers of hospitals met the stringent conditions laid down by the DoH in order to become independent trusts. GPs before becoming 'fund-holding' practices had also to meet certain standards including sufficient numbers of patients to sustain an adequate range of budgeted services (at first set at 11 000, later reduced to 9000).

In practice, numbers opting out have been small. In the months following the publication of the White Paper in 1989, referenda held in many leading hospitals on whether to 'opt-out' revealed deep divisions between their newly appointed general managers and the point of delivery staff led, in many cases, by consultants. Nevertheless advocates of the 'internal market' see the process as irrevocable. The number of 'independent' hospitals and GPs need only reach a relatively low critical mass to sustain internal market pressures within the NHS. Coping with the pressures derived from the internal mixed economy is seen to provide the drive needed for efficiency within RHAs, DHAs and FHSAs.

Opposition has come from at least three differing perspectives. Firstly, there is a broadly based fear of 'managerialism' which is echoed throughout this volume but is most clearly articulated by Cox in Chapter 2. This is directed at the inappropriateness of scientific management, or the imposition of quantitatively based measurement and control, in the delivery of a critically personal service.

Secondly, there are the opponents of the use of market-threats to introduce managerial reform. These can be seen as further dividing into two distinctive groups. First there are the technical critics who recognize the appalling confusion of contradictory information bases and information systems that exist within the NHS and regard the objectives of the Act as unattainable within the short term. Some see the introduction of 'market forces' as combining with short deadlines to compound the present administrative problems through forcing the adoption of a variety of readily available information technologies (IT) (see Chapter 9).

Another, possibly more important, source of opposition to the market mechanism derives from a political belief that health care is a basic personal and communal need and is best controlled through the medium of elected authorities. It must, however, be noted that neither political nor technical opponents of the 1990 reforms discount the necessity for managerial reform. Indeed, the proposals advanced by the Labour Party contain a necessity for planned budgeting and offer incentives for outperforming these targets (*A Fresh Start for Health*, 1990). There appears, then, to be a recognition across all parts of the political spectrum that government attempts at administrative innovation over the last quarter century have not brought adaptation or flexibility in service sufficient to meet changing social priorities.

The visible hand of caring

There is, indeed, an apparent paradox present in the fact that by any objective comparison of successful innovation in product or process, the performance of the health care sector in the UK must rank highly relative to all other forms of service delivery, and, more especially, with innovation in the manufacturing industries. Few other sectors of the UK economy can compare with the ability of the NHS to successfully implement new forms of service at a so-called 'world class' level. It might appear that its very success has contributed to its present embarrassment. One explanation for the prolonged and worsening financial problems of the NHS is that the pace of development and deployment of new materials and equipment in the diagnosis and treatment of human ailments has outrun the ability of the rest of the economy to pay. Taken together with their success in the prolongation of human life and control over birth, health carers might be seen to have shaped the nature of a burgeoning high-cost, labour-intensive marketplace. Furthermore, their apparent success in delivering ever more effective products has raised consumer expectations and has brought about an apparently limitless propensity to consume health care.

Without the constraint of price competition the question of responsibility for adjudging the allocation of resources to meet this rising tide of generated needs has inevitably become an issue in UK national politics. From the passing of the Poor Law (1834) the role of the state as agent of the consuming public has steadily increased. Nor is this peculiar to the UK. In most industrialized countries, including the USA, the state is a major direct provider of resources as well as acting indirectly as a regulator of the market and accreditor of service providers and suppliers. At the same time, the role of agent in determining the best interests of the individual in need has largely resided with the physician-surgeon. In few other societal contexts does either a service provider or a state agency seek such power over the welfare of the individual citizen. In few other fields do suppliers enjoy monopoly rents created by government sponsorship and the accreditation accorded to the health care profession and the producers of drugs and medical equipment.

The existence of the 'visible hand' of government in the moulding of consumer choices inevitably leads to debate which, in liberal democracies, is itself a source of costly delay (Olson, 1982; Stocking, 1985). The main elements of this debate are examined in Chapter 2 by Cox. It is a debate which, again, is not unique to the UK. Even in the USA, modes of financing health care in a way that would provide an effective service to *all* sections of the community are the continuing subject of fierce debate and political division (Aaron and Schwartz, 1985; Jonas and Rosenberg, 1986). Where, as in the UK, the state has taken on the major role of resource-provider, as well as regulator and accreditor of the service provider, the evolution of the system has been marked by a series of parliamentary interventions in attempts at more effective solutions. It would be possible to attribute many of the present difficulties in the management of the NHS to the *ad hoc* nature of these interventions and to the pragmatic nature in which directions have been determined by the DoH (formerly

incorporating Social Services, the DHSS) and by a succession of government ministers. The lack of coherent strategic direction or of a clear
statement of principles and objectives has been commented on by each
would-be reformist inquiry from 1972 through to 1979 and, finally, in the
Review of NHS Management conducted by Lord Griffiths (then Mr Roy
Griffiths), an executive from a supermarket chain in 1983 (DHSS, 1983).
The changes that have resulted have often been seen to be more procedural
than substantive and to have reinforced the scepticism displayed towards
managers by carers, particularly among doctors and nurses.

Operational fragmentation versus occupational unity

It would be equally possible to suggest that the problems of the NHS are
not ones of top-level policy but rather reflect the quality of NHS management at local level. This may be seen as lacking in the necessary skills and
authority to implement DHSS policy or to initiate local administrative
reform. In each of the Parliamentary Reports and White Papers concern
has been expressed for managerial structures and competencies. During
the 1970s the lack of specialist expertise among national DHSS administrators and local RHAs drew constant criticism. This was an era described by
Klein (1983) as commencing in a spirit of technocratic idealism. There was
a new sense of rational design in the creation of administrative structures
and in the search for economies of scale and scope within the provision of
public services generally.

In the 1974 reforms, there was also an attempt to enfranchise medical
staff, or perhaps more accurately, to co-opt them into the process of
management through their incorporation into so-called 'teams' at each
level of decision-making within the NHS. By the end of the decade these
attempts, according to the same author, had declined into the 'politics of
disillusionment'. Joint decision-making between administrators and professional service providers had led to a slowing rather than quickening of
change in NHS reforms. At national and regional level, the ambiguity that
surrounded the process of communal goal-setting over the period of the
1950s and 1960s had, by that time, given way to the harsh priorities of a
national economy in crisis. In a service in which 80% of the costs derive
from wages and salaries, the financial cuts instituted in the 1970s fed
directly into labour unrest and further eroded the already declining basis of
altruism that had been a feature of staff commitment from the early days
of the NHS.

The same drive for economy brought a return to managerialism as the
basis for reform during the 1980s. The Körner Committee was brought
into being by the minister to provide advice on suitable means of creating
standardized forms of management information (Körner, 1982, 1983). Roy
Griffiths recommended a greater concentration of authority in general
manager positions at all levels of the NHS (DHSS, 1983), an apparent

contradiction of the prevailing 'team' principle. If the adoption of the latter proposal in the following year was intended to attract more professionally educated personnel from outside the NHS into the new positions it clearly failed since most were internal appointments (Alleway, 1986). Perhaps because of this, as well as because of a multitude of contributory obstacles, the adoption of standardized information systems, even within the most localized of administrative areas, the DHA, has appeared to many observers, including contributors to this volume, to be agonizingly slow.

In the early 1980s, Klein (1983) had attributed managerial inertia to the 'politics of organisational stasis'. He traces this condition back to the roots of the NHS, in the compromises between government and the various branches of the medical profession that made the NHS possible in the first place. The key factor underpinning this compromise was the creation of a viable basis for consensus in operational goals. This was achieved but at a cost of introducing into the management of the service a 'bias towards inertia' (Klein, 1983, p. 58). The medical profession has largely succeeded in defining certain areas as out of bounds to non-professionals; that is to managers (Klein, 1983, p. 57),

> its power lay ... in shaping the perceptions of policy problems – of incorporating a professional bias into the assumptive world of the policy-makers. While it did not dominate the NHS in terms of getting what it wanted in a positive sense, it did succeed in asserting its right of veto in specific policy spheres ... from being the main opponents of the NHS, the doctors had in effect become the strongest force for the *status quo*.

It would be only a little exaggerated to suggest that most of government interventions in the post-War period have been attempts to redress this balance of power away from that accorded doctors in the design of the original NHS structure. Yet for many commentators it has appeared as if 'they are administering history ... rather than planning for the future' (Day and Klein, 1983). These authors see the parallel structure of representation and consultation in which the collective views of doctors are expressed variously by the Royal Colleges of Medicine and by the British Medical Association (BMA) as part of the price paid by the, then, Minister of Health, Aneurin Bevan, for the support of these bodies in the foundation of the NHS.

Possibly this view discounts both the longevity and universality of the influence exercised by doctors within *all* societies. With the possible exception of the legal professions, few groups have been so consistently successful in bringing pressure on the UK parliamentary process as those of the medical profession (Parry and Parry, 1976). Furthermore, their influence has extended to shaping the workplace roles and market status accorded by the state to almost all other occupational interests that contribute to the hierarchy of skills and authority which make up the NHS (Larkin, 1983).

Two studies in this volume illustrate the continued efficacy of the efforts of
community physicians (GPs) in maintaining their occupational boundaries.
In Chapter 6, Greenfield writes an optimistic account of the growing
diagnostic role of the nurse in general practice. In Chapter 7, Blenkinsopp
suggests that, within the constraints of the statutory limits set upon their
diagnostic activities, community pharmacists have been able to expand the
scope of their services. These cases demonstrate both the possible scope
for delegation of duties presently reserved exclusively for accredited physicians and, by the very scarcity of these examples of devolution, the
national influence of medical representation.

It might even be said that the structures and models of service delivery
that were articulated in the Health Service Act (1948) were little more than
the institutional enshrinement of the principles of occupational authority
sought after by the Royal Colleges for nearly two centuries. To do so
would be to exaggerate the opportunistic pragmatism that has characterized the, very British, manner in which medical interests have evolved,
have gained Royal sponsorship and have become the accredited custodians
of medical knowledge within our national society. Indeed it may be suggested that a lack of coherent strategy for health care management is
as characteristic of the stances taken by the Royal Colleges and of the
BMA, as of the ministry itself. The collective purposes of the former have
focussed primarily upon the maintenance of the individual status and
authority of each of their members within the carer–patient relationship.
In these circumstances, any collective attempt to define community need
taken by representatives of the profession qua profession contains the risk
of undermining the scope for personal judgement by its individual members. Such attempts have therefore only rarely, and somewhat tardily,
been undertaken. In other words these professional interest associations
have, by their very nature, been defensive rather than initiating bodies. At
the same time the emphasis placed on the defence of the individual autonomy of their members in the task situation has tended to bias their responses towards encouraging a *curative* approach to health care management
in which the doctor has retained his or her personal scope for judgement
rather than a *preventative* or community-based perspective. This is a perspective which the new contracts offered to the profession by the DoH evidently seeks to redress (see Bryden's analysis in Chapter 5).

The retention of a wide area of medical authority has evidently cut
across all regulatory or procedural controls required for the coordination
and direction of a complex administrative bureaucracy like a District
Hospital. The nature of professional agency claimed by each doctor
requires him or her to attempt to prescribe whatever is considered best for
the treatment of a client. Thus doctors, and more particularly consultants
within whose province lies the most capital intensive areas of health care
provision, carry considerable power to determine the eventual allocation,
or realized demand, for NHS resources. As many critics have suggested,
the shape of NHS health care services is determined by the aggregate of

clinical decisions of individual consultants. This is particularly brought out in the analysis of the doctor's position in the distribution of pharmaceutical products presented in Chapter 3.

Complementaries and contradictions

The most quotable comment of the Griffiths Report must be the suggestion that 'if Florence Nightingale were carrying her lamp through the NHS today she would almost certainly be searching for the people in charge' (DHSS, 1983). In practice, organizational theorists have been carrying lamps through hospitals and health care organizations generally for decades in an attempt to understand the bifurcated nature of their authority structures (Gordon, 1962). Mintzberg (1982) has described them as the archetypical professional-bureaucracy in which administrators defer to service deliverers in matters concerning clients but draw their own influence from their separate relationship with resource providers such as the state, private insurance companies and charitable foundations.

It may be thought that this description of a relative evenness in the balance of power between complementary functions is a fairly simplistic one. It is, however, drawn from a North American context in which managers derive considerable power from their ability as fund-raisers. As such it may be seen as a model to which the drafters of the 1990 Act aspire. Mintzberg recognizes the potential conflicts that can surface in this bifurcated-authority system but seems to rely on the influence of market forces, through insurance payments, or of external arbitration, through state intervention, to break deadlocks between bureaucrats and professionals. Strauss *et al.* (1963), by contrast, spoke of the constant 'negotiation of order' within US hospital settings made up of numerous competing hierarchies of specialist and support staff. This latter description is reflected in the various terms that have been used to label health care organizations as 'polyarchies', 'heteroarchies', or, more simply, as higher-order variations on craft-administrative systems (Anthony, 1989).

It is perhaps worth noting the universality of the tensions being analysed in these studies of the organization of health care delivery, and the fact that the most notable of the latter works derive not from the NHS, but from the so-called market-based systems of North America. While the mode of state regulation or active involvement in the provision of health care systems does have an effect on their administrative structures from one country to another, there is a remarkable similarity in the workplace organization of care delivery and the strength of occupational identity between those involved in its delivery (Child and Loveridge, 1990). The former appear most often to be divided locally by specialized departmental hierarchies, but these are conjoined across hospitals or localities by stongly stratified occupational loyalties. As a result of this cross-fractionation of interest boundaries, the informally negotiated norms of the workgroup take on a particular significance in the manner observed by Strauss.

An understanding of these local work norms is essential to the effective operations of groups that have to meet crisis conditions within their task environment, often without prior warning (Harvey, 1985). Role adaptations are immensely varied within local configurations of norms. These are often translated into the local structures and processes of formal administration. For example, the minutiae involved in passing a patient from one department to another often make use of quite different pro-forma comparing one hospital with another only a few miles distant. Potential savings from economies of scale stemming from the standard-ization of routinized information processing are disregarded even in areas of the most apparently mundane activities. Perhaps more important are the effects of such variety on the operational effectiveness of a *national* service in respect to both epidemiological research and its ability to under-stand and cope with anything other than local crises.

Nurses, who comprise the largest single occupational group in health care, tend to become the repositories and guardians of local custom and practice. They are the preservers of order around the patient treatment regime as well as the principal care deliverers (Salvage, 1985). As a consequence they, together with medical secretaries, appear as conflict managers *par excellence* (Evers, 1976). Their attitudes often display a con-servatism and desire to retain a *status quo*. These may in fact reflect a situation in which there exists only a precarious and dynamic equilibrium between the pressing demands of multifarious specialist service providers laying claim to domain over the patient's body and the technology used to treat it. Both Sharifi (Chapter 13) and Grieco (Chapter 14) describe how local groups, and more particularly nursing officers, shaped the design of new hospitals through the timing and targeting of their interventions in ways that avoided overt confrontations with medical authority. Therefore, to characterize attitudes of this, or any other occupational group, as 'conservative' in the conventional use of the term, or to regard these locally fragmented cultures as evidence of organizational lethargy, would be to show a dangerous disregard for the underlying dynamics that hold the care delivery system in place. Furthermore, such an assumed lethargy might lead to a disregard for the essentially individualistic context that induces the speed of innovation in medical diagnosis and practice. The idiosyncratic nature of the process has caused many observers to criticize both its efficacy and its 'scientific' objectivity. It is clear that changes in health care practice that do *not* focus on the biomedical paradigm that frames the boundaries of professional contest are likely to be ignored or neglected by doctors. Georgopoulos' (1982) study of the uptake of new knowledge in US hospitals serves to affirm that a similar bias in innovation diffusion exists in that country's health care delivery system. New forms of diagnosis and treatment derive as much from the individualistic contest for professional recognition and prestige as from any spirit of altruism. This is well illustrated by Shaw's analysis of the conduit for technological innovation in clinical equipment provided by the 'invisible college' of medical consultants set out in Chapter 8.

Organizational changes designed to correct the bias outlined above have, therefore, to be seen as prejudicing the social or relational system from which it springs. Starkey (Chapter 4) sees the changing contractual terms of consultants as indicating just such a threat to their autonomy. Yet there is little in the recent history of UK commerce and manufacturing to suggest that there exist readily available alternative models of the successful management of research and development (R & D) that can be easily transposed into this, the largest single centralized enterprise in Europe.

The irresistible wave of Thatcherism?

The minister and DoH (formerly the DHSS) have, in the past, attempted three models of bringing about changes in administrative policy and practice. The first is that of setting up bodies of inquiry having status ranging from that of Royal Commission to that of internal DoH working party. Acting on reports from such bodies may require the minister to seek an Act of Parliament as in the case of the changes stemming from the 1989 White Paper *Working for Patients* which passed into law in June 1990. An example of an internally generated reform was the creation of the nurse-manager grades following the Salmon Report of 1972. However the most drastic change to be implemented in this manner was the series of measures by which responsibility for the general management of resources at the level of individual hospitals, districts, regions and at the level of the NHS itself was, in 1984, passed to executives with direct responsibility to boards at each level appointed through the minister personally.

The more diffused mode in which the DoH seeks to exercise influence is through formal circulars offering guides to good practice issued on a regular basis which, like the Highway Code, do not have the immediate force of law, but may be quoted in cases of administrative negligence. In the case of medical, technological or administrative changes, a system of prototyping new developments has been evolved since the early days of the NHS. This involves the establishment of a number of pilot schemes that are generously funded over a trial period of perhaps seven years, usually in a manner that is shared with the RHAs and DHAs to whose charge the experiment eventually reverts. In this manner it is hoped that exemplars of the latest practice may be set, often in a way that allows other local authorities a choice between different systems included in the pilot.

Historically, it cannot be said that, however admirable these modes of change management might appear in the pluralistic context of the NHS, the process has proven successful in fostering speedy adoption. The intense 'not-invented-here' spirit in which administrators and health care managers have tended to respond to an innovation in other regions or districts seems often to have a counteractive effect on its diffusion. However it was in the latter mode that the DoH attempted to gain acceptance for the crucial second component of the Griffiths reforms – that of the computerization of management budgeting. The focus of this strategy was that of devolving the responsibility of maintaining budgets to the point of service delivery. The philosophy behind the formulation of this strategy is discussed by Coombs and Cooper in Chapter 9. A number of trial sites were agreed for the introduction of clinical budgeting into large hospitals. These exercises could be seen to have been an attempt to co-opt clinicians into the managerial process by acknowledging their specialist department as a separate cost centre. Each centre was evaluated through an agreed measure of its output performance in providing patient care. The aim was to convert doctors into resource managers who would receive rapid feedback concerning the resource consequences of their operational decisions and be constrained by this information in future decisions. Many early volunteers reported favourably on their experiences (one hospital actually appointed full-time departmental 'business' managers).

Nevertheless, the initiative might well have lingered on as one of the diverse portfolios of such experiments in new management information systems (MIS), together with their associated national and regional agencies, that have come into being over the last 20 years with little more than an isolated localized impact. The manner in which early efforts at introducing MIS met with varied responses is described in Chapter 10 by Dent *et al*. However, the tidal wave of Thatcherite reform impelled its incorporation within the much more ambitious Resource Management Initiative of November 1986, currently aimed at involving 250 hospitals by the mid-1990s. When set against the total number of hospital units in the country (over 2000) the goal still appears unambitious.

The primary problem remains that identified by Körner, and numerous previous inquiries – that of lack of standardized cost and performance data with which to monitor the overall performance of the NHS. Behind this problem lies the deeper one of the incipient attachment of actors to a diversity of highly localized procedures and practices encapsulated in both informal custom and practice and the minutiae of multiple complex bureaucracies.

The White Paper of January 1989 represented the third, and what was hoped to be the decisive element in bringing about structural reform in the NHS. This involved the creation of an 'internal' market for services on the basis of a contest between hospital units for client custom as represented through the agency of primary carers, that is through GPs. The allocation of funding was to remain with RHAs and DHAs but was to be guided by the choices of GPs in relation to the price/value offers made by hospital consultants and within the constraints set by the GP's own budget. This in turn was to be, and now is, set in relation to a series of prices allocated by the government in relation to their conception of community priorities as well as on the number of patients served by each GP. Hospitals could if they so wished, become financially autonomous through applying to the minister for permission to become self-governing trusts.

Ultimately, it was not envisaged that the state would lose its role as the principal resource provider. One can perhaps be excused for discerning in the White Paper and the 1990 Act a political shift in interest away from management budgeting *per se* to internal markets (Pollitt *et al.*, 1988, p. 232). The aim is to encourage competition for scarce resources and the diversification of revenue sources. A new breed of entrepreneurial manager competes among itself to generate and to capture resources. The rationale for an increased focus on competition is that recourse to a market for resources throws into sharp relief 'the issues of cost and quality, the need to be explicit about standards of care and the need for good financial information' (Drummond and Maynard, 1988, p. 69). The use of a market for services facilitates cost-effective exchange by providing a 'mechanism whereby buyers and sellers exchange goods and services, using prices as signals to inform exchange' (Drummond and Maynard, 1988, p. 60).

Recourse to market mechanisms has already led to a contracting out of ancillary services such as catering and cleaning to private firms and of operations to private hospitals. Paralleling this development is the growth in use of private medical insurance, for which there has been a trebling in numbers since 1979. Right-wing critics of the NHS see privatization as the best means of increasing efficient use of resources rather than making small but politically unpopular financial gains through increases in costs for services to patients (Pirie, 1988).

The model of control that has emerged from this debate contains many of the 'tight–loose' characteristics of the so-called 'flexible-firm' (Peters and Waterman, 1982; Atkinson, 1985). The centre retains ultimate control over the allocation of strategic resources but is guided in its actions by operational choices made at the periphery in response to market demand. Supporting this initiative there has been a determined effort to inject managerial expertise into strategic decision making at national, regional, area and community (FHSA) levels of the NHS. It was also the publicly expressed view of the Government, as described in the White Paper's title, that greater consumer choice would break the power of local and occupational monopoly. The agent chosen to carry out this mission was not the consumer personally, but members of that part of the medical profession that had, since the middle of the last century, been regarded as being of lesser status – the GPs. This is the agency responsibility embraced enthusiastically by Bryden (Chapter 5) in what may currently be considered a somewhat unrepresentative GP response.

In many ways, the White Paper and the Act that came into being in mid-1990 showed considerable political ingenuity in dividing the loyalties of the professions while accomplishing many of the perceived needs of central planning. Not least among these was the pressure for the introduction of standardized MIS for the purposes of controlling costs and evaluating comparative performance within the internal market. Against this there may be said to exist all of the obstacles to change that have previously stood in the way of such managerial reforms. Thus the aim of installing standardized information systems over the period of three to five years allowed for the changes have been seen as an impossible one and therefore as a reason for rejecting the whole internal market concept. (BMA statements May/June 1990, reported in *Pulse* (1990)).

More fundamental, however, is the opposition inspired by a fear that the spirit of competition may prove all too effective in changing practitioner and consumer motives. This is most often expressed in the belief that the growing use of private health care facilities will accelerate either because individual patients will opt out of remaining NHS hospitals or because private care providers will prove more cost-effective in the 'soft' sectors of the market and gain a significant proportion of the more profitable sub-contracts from RHAs or DHAs (*Pulse*, 1990). Perhaps a more insidious effect on the present basis of service provision might stem from changes in the behaviour of individual providers of care service towards becoming more opportunistic in their pursuit of market recognition and financial rewards. There is some evidence that a movement in this direction could be found in the choice of patients made by GPs in the months following the introduction of selective payments in 1990.

Almost certainly the competition by hospitals to obtain or retain the services of key medical specialists will express itself in a growing disparity between consultants' salaries and also in the allocation of capital investment required to provide specialists with sufficient new equipment to attract their loyalty. (Indeed the latter may become the principal tie to one place of work for a peripatetic consultant in high demand across several contractors.) This may lead to even greater distortions than those present in the previously existing contest between occupational interests within a state bureaucracy. Thus, say critics, the fundamental need for regulation and direction by the state will not disappear any more than it has in any other industrialized country. Its solution could only lie in fundamental changes in the division of labour within the practice of health care delivery. Ultimately the growing encroachment of managerial control may succeed in bringing that about but so far changes in occupational hierarchies remain slight compared to innovation in the rest of the world outside of health care.

Technological innovation in the NHS

A major force in the creation of new occupations in the NHS has been technological innovation. As has been commented upon previously, technological innovation has found a more willing reception in the service among medical professionals than major administrative reforms. The contribution that new technology has made to the improvement of clinical performance can hardly be contested. The diffusion of such technological innovations in the NHS can be seen to follow two main paths. The first is that, as described earlier, of top-down strategic initiatives pursued in a number of ways but mostly by the DoH circular or aid to regions or districts in establishing exemplar sites for prototyping the new practice. The second, and hitherto more powerful one (described by Shaw in Chapter 8), the force of occupational emulation, emphasizes the importance of the medical profession in the horizontal diffusion of clinical innovation. When set against the latter's influence in the generation and recognition of para-medical and support services at the point of production, the doctors' control over operational technology can be seen to be central to their continued status and authority.

As might be expected, the historical focus of clinical innovation has been in practices within hospitals. It is there that most new capital formation has taken place rather than in the practice of community medicine: indeed as Vann-Wye (Chapter 12) and others point out, hospital design has played a key historical role in the working out of professional control strategies. Investment in hospital buildings represents not simply one of the largest portions of NHS investment but also in national public investment overall. While the ideas of architects and planners have clearly shaped the direction of this investment, Vann-Wye alleges (Chapter 12) that the medical paradigm has never been seriously challenged by these more immediate contributions to hospital design.

An equally expensive and influential investment in new technology has been that in information technology (IT). The most overt articulation of an IT strategy in the NHS has been that already described above in respect to MIS. There can be little doubt, however, that the earliest and by far the greatest application of microelectronic devices has been in clinical diagnosis and treatment. The first major scientific meeting devoted to the prospects of using the computer in clinical health care was held in New York in January 1959 (Reiser, 1978). Two features of the computer particularly captivated physicians: its capacity to store information and its ability to search for and establish complicated relationships within the data. The field was already undergoing a crisis because of the mounting amount of data required to keep up with the expanding funds of knowledge together with the difficulty of incorporating the latter into a single complete diagnosis. The computer also helped to integrate into medical practice the numerous electro-mechanical devices designed to continuously monitor the physiological condition of the body. The use of semiconductors began in the 1950s, and by the 1960s mainframe computers were widely used in clinical scanning and monitoring. The invention of microprocessors in the 1970s heralded a surge in the use of automated bed-side equipment and the utilization of personal computers for recording information by hospital doctors and for producing preprogramed instructions for patient treatment to be utilized by nursing staff.

There was initially a widespread suspicion of computer engineering in the medical profession, and, indeed, its members are still divided in their attitudes toward the growing substitution of machines for nurses in bed-side diagnosis and treatment, particularly in the operating theatre. Among the foremost fears expressed at the time was that medical diagnosis could actually be so programed as to leave little room for the physician's judgement. Since the computer could analyse much more data more rigorously than the human mind the *British Medical Journal* even forecast a role for the doctor as a 'sort of machine minder' (Reiser, 1978, p. 223).

However, as Rogers (1983) has suggested, the pioneers of an innovation are likely to be those who have most need for it and with whose existing practices it proves most compatible. These were in areas of scanning, testing and monitoring of clinical samples. Not only were machine enthusiasts likely to be found in these activities, but within the annual round of hospital bids for new capital equipment, departmental heads in these areas were able to make a convincing case for integrating their existing administrative activities and so achieving economies of scale through the purchase of a computer.

More recently, however, new technology has become *a crucial*, if not *the crucial* variable, in government attempts to reform the NHS, and IT has become increasingly central to the direction of government strategy. IT is the key to the dissemination of MIS. Post-Griffiths, the principal means of involving clinicians more closely in the management process have focussed on the integration of new systems of management budgeting with the attempted measurement of output performance in terms of patient care. The aim is to turn doctors into resource managers with access to rapid personal feedback concerning the resource consequences of their day-to-day activities. Here the role of new technology is likely to be crucial. Innovations in IT offer radical new organizational possibilities. New technologies have 'changed the economic cost-benefit balance in favour of greatly enlarging the information-processing capabilities of codified/formalized information and its wider diffusion' (Child, 1987, p. 43). Child highlights, in particular, the possibilities of facilitating a trend towards various kinds of external transactions and a move away from wholly internal transactions as a way of reducing costs and managing risk in an uncertain environment.

IT in the administration of UK health care had its formal initiation in the 1960s with a DHSS initiative following the Flowers Report. It offered financial technical support to RHAs in establishing mainframe services for their own use and that of Area and District Authorities. This was followed by a number of specific attempts to establish prototypes in MIS. In 1968, the DHSS attempted to initiate a series of prototypes in the use of computerized patient administrative systems (PAS). There was little response but two hospitals in the West Midlands Region became the sites of first experiments. In 1970, North Staffordshire Royal Infirmary in Stoke-on-Trent adopted a whole hospital admissions system and Queen Elizabeth

Hospital in Birmingham, a ward based and laboratory system. This was a significant event which, like many other potentially contentious initiatives, remained largely isolated to the progenitors in its effects after the five-year trial period was up.

Potentially PAS can be seen as a bridge between the needs of logistical management in allocating bed-units (including staffing, etc.) to patients, or to matching anticipated flows of patients to stocks of bed-units, and the needs of clinical staff for the personal medical histories of those patients. This junction is one of the most critical in the hospital system, since it brings together, on an equal footing, the separate needs of the administration and the clinician. Dependent upon the programming of this combination of data, both parties might have equal access to the information required by, and the recorded judgements of, the other.

Needless to say, the boundaries to these two bodies of knowledge that had been built up socially over several centuries were not usually easily transgressed through the limited techniques of computer programers. However, if the task autonomy of the doctors (how they performed) was to remain little affected by PAS, the procedural control over their timing (when they performed) was brought under severe questioning by the new system (see Grieco, Chapter 14). Without wishing to exaggerate the importance of the early prototypes, it is interesting to note that the Queen Elizabeth Hospital, which placed an emphasis on *clinically* relevant information, seemed to generate less internal conflict than that of the other pioneer, Stoke Infirmary, which attempted to match the timing of consultant *availability* to that of patient flows. Several contributors to this volume return to this theme of the politicality of decisions concerning the autonomy of care deliverers.

During the 1980s, under pressure from the reports of the Steering Group on Health Services Information (chaired by Edith Körner), some RHAs adopted rolling plans for the implementation of PAS systems throughout their areas. These reports were directed at the increased systemization and standardization of MIS at all levels of the NHS in the manner described by Dent *et al.* in Chapter 10. The needs of hospital administration were regarded as particularly urgent because of their vast use of resources in the treatment of a minority of severely ill patients. However, community health systems were also being designed in increasing numbers of cities and towns. GPs were perhaps among the most reluctant adopters but in response to the inducements of two major pharmaceutical manufacturers, the slow diffusion of GP systems began in the latter part of the decade. Taken together with the more rapid adoption of Accident and Emergency (A & E) systems, the theoretical potential for networking across local health care systems – primary and secondary – and even across the national system has become increasingly evident by the 1990s.

Although segmented, the overall market for IT provided by the NHS is one of the greatest in the world. Small wonder then that all major computer manufacturers have specialized divisions or branches marketing their health administrative systems. At the beginning of the 1990s, nearly 300 UK-based bespoke designer computer consultants exist in the field. Given the short timespan allowed before the new legislation following on the 1989 White Paper placed hospitals on a competitive footing, and created conditions in which large GP practices could be run as businesses, the scramble to get IT systems in place has probably created as much differentiation in component design as it has common standards. Given also the problem of integrating the diverse activities of the NHS, it is not surprising that the most available software systems are those based on conventional accountancy or resource planning models of a relatively limited kind. As Coombs and Cooper suggest (Chapter 9) these systems contain little acknowledgement of the underlying values and patterns of activity within health care management. On the other hand, the devolution of budgetary control to local units brought about by the 1990 Act and the pre-existing experiments in clinical budgeting that followed the Griffiths Report, indicate a very different mode and style of management control may be about to emerge. This is intended to involve the creation of standard means of activity-measurement and cost-allocation systems across hospital departments and community health services. By means of these standards the local hierarchies of costs and estimated benefits linked to the treatment of ailments should, theoretically, be comparable. Thus the price signals charged by units in local markets could be related to resources available publicly at national level.

Coordinating the politics of change

Situations of radical, structural change re-open access to resources control and, indeed, can lead to the redefinition of what are considered as resources in the pursuit of new strategies. In the attempts being made by care deliverers and by delivery managers to interpret the operational meaning of the 1990 Act new theories and new practices will be discovered in a situation in which many of the old procedural prompts will no longer be available from RHAs and DHAs and in which, therefore, the informal, 'custom-and-practice' modes of responding will be equally redundant.

In a comparison of innovation across European health care services (Child and Loveridge, 1990), conflict was most present in the UK cases. In Chapter 11, Ahmad describes a case history in the engagement of the author, a medical consultant, with general management in conflict over the design of a MIS. For the adoption and commissioning of MIS, PAS or any other major administrative IT project, the process is one in which the manager must bring together a series of working parties involving the 'team' of senior medical, nursing and other specialist officers, as well as 'experts' from regional and district computer services. The case has to be made, and remade, for the project in 'studies' and 'reports' of an entirely different nature to that of the independent bid for funds from a medical departmental head. In Chapter 13, Sharifi describes this process in relation to the commissioning of a new hospital.

In all of this, the manager has often to be the initiator of change, as well as its orchestrator. The commissioning and routinization of the change is long, drawn out and marked by incidents such as refusals by medical secretaries to collaborate in the revelation of their boss's waiting lists or pattern of appointments. Admission of error by any one of the parties is equally delayed and 'problems', therefore, difficult to isolate. This is a situation in which the external management consultant or systems designer has become an increasingly prevalent actor as an uninvolved judge of the parties' needs rather than as a conciliator of existing needs. The amendment on total redesign of IT systems appears to take place very frequently. This often seems to be because the computerized system itself was designed around a poor understanding of the actual workings of care delivery in a given situation, being often modelled on an overseas prototype. Of itself, the political tension existing between competing groups within the domestic systems has not provided the best basis for arriving at a concurrence with the needs of the collectivity when specifying the client brief for the systems designer. Such exercises have often been enormously expensive in terms of the later operation of the system and, even more so, in lost opportunity.

Clearly a key skill in effective general management is that of managing the political tensions of an organization comprised of competing interest groups (Wrapp, 1967). The oppositional interests contained in professional bodies have created an essentially federal process of health care delivery. In this sense no health care management system in the world comprises a normal organizational hierarchy. In such a situation of contested authority, the general manager who hopes to be able to steer the process of strategic decision-making must possess sufficient expertise in the design and maintenance of overall organizational systems to be able to make a unique contribution to this process. There is no basis in research for believing that either formal authority or social skills will suffice as grounds for long-term leadership in even the most stable of operating environments.

The formal position of the general manager within the new NHS structure provides the occupant with the opportunity to analyse the system in its total context and to create strategic options which extend beyond the localized concerns of clinicians, GPs and other care deliverers. The potential leverage provided by the formal authority given to general management in the Act has to be transformed into actual strategic influence through educated analysis and an ability to persuade others of its appropriateness as a basis for action.

It is an open question as to whether sufficient capabilities yet exist within the NHS. Current recruits to general management positions have displayed a remarkable continuity with previous sources of NHS administrators. There could, however, be a rapid opening up of the labour market in the face of cut-backs in other areas of service employment and increases in the financial inducements offered to general managers within the NHS. In the light of the historic position held by members of the medical and nursing professions within the management of health care it would, perhaps, be a rash prophet who discounted the role of the doctor or nurse as general manager in the new NHS in spite of continued remonstrations by their Royal Colleges.

Conclusion

Portentous statements on the future provision of this life-sustaining service have been the stuff of politics since the emergence of a collective conscience in Western industrial societies during the last century. Given the vocational controls over service delivery, what has yet to be discovered is an entirely effective and economic way to manage the links that conjoin the various caring services. This is a matter that divides academic observers as much as politicians. On one hand, there are those who see moral commitment as the only possible binding force. Others would reduce all caring action to a set of utilitarian cyphers. Information technology provides a vehicle for an enormous extension of strategic choice based on a variety of models for service delivery. In France, for example, we have the 'smart card' voucher introduced in the late 1980s which allows the individual client enormous choice within an electronic marketplace served by both the state and by private finance. In Scandinavia there are the publicly orchestrated but regionally decentralized systems of health care. Both provide possible models towards which the UK system might develop under the pressures of internal contest.

What has been lacking in the past history of the NHS is any sense of systemic logic along which progress could be made, incrementally, but with a discernible pattern of intent. The confusion that has resulted has often been described as 'pluralism'. It never was, because not all parties had the same basis to influence the system and, ultimately, the stalemate that resulted did nothing to emancipate the patient. In the new arrangements, the GP has once more become the patient's champion. Whether these primary carers are able to utilize their power of choice effectively will depend on their capabilities as managers of markets as well as within their practice hierarchies. Enthoven, the progenitor of the internal market concept believes these skills to be presently lacking among UK GPs (*The Independent*, 26 January 1991, p. 8). Perhaps equally important to the future of a national service is the capability of the general managers at all levels of the service to take full advantage of information technology in the creation and coordination of strategic direction. Ultimately, however, the ability of managers to create a cultural climate in which loyalty to the operational unit complements and reinforces a prior moral attachment to occupational vocation among carers will remain important to the quality of service received by the client. If the experiences of the last 20 years have taught UK business executives anything at all, it must be that competition at the end of the twentieth century is based primarily on quality of service and not simply on price.

References

Aaron, H.J. and Schwartz, W.B. (1985) Hospital cost control: a bitter pill to swallow. *Harvard Business Review*, **64**, March–April, 160–7.

Alleway, L. (1986) Why Mr Paige couldn't manage. *Nursing Times*, 2 July, 16–17.

Anthony, P. (1989) Managerial roles and relationships: the impact of the Griffiths Report, *Meeting the Challenge of Health Service Management: UK and Canadian Experiences*, Canada House, London, 10 January.

Atkinson, J. (1985) *Flexibility, Uncertainty, and Manpower Management*. Brighton: Institute of Manpower Studies.

Child, J. (1987) Information technology, organization and the response to strategic challenges. *California Management Review*, Fall, 33–50.

Child, J. and Loveridge, R. (1990) *Information Technology in European Services*. Oxford: Basil Blackwell.

Day, P. and Klein, K. (1983) The mobilisation of consent versus the management of conflict: decoding the Griffiths Report. *British Medical Journal*, **287**, 1813–16.

Department of Health and Social Security (1983) *NHS Management Inquiry (The Griffiths Report)*. London: DHSS.

Drummond, M. and Maynard, A. (1988) Efficiency in the National Health Service: lessons from abroad. *Health Policy*, **9**, 59–74.

Enthoven, A. (1985) *Reflections on the Management of the National Health Service*. London: Nuffield Provincial Hospitals Trust.

Evers, H. (1976) The role of the medical secretary. Aston Management Centre Working Paper No. 58.

Georgopoulos, B.S. (1982) Organizational rationality, medicine, and the use of new knowledge in American hospitals. *Hospital and Health Services Administration*, **27**, 34–56.

Gordon, P.J. (1962) The top management triangle in voluntary hospitals. I and II. *Journal of the Academy of Management*, **4**, 205–214; **5**, 66–75.

Grinyer, P.H. and Spender, J.C. (1979) *Turnaround – Managerial Recipes for Corporate Success*. London: Associated Business Press.

Harvey, J. (1985) Living between life and death. *New Society*, 8 November, 233–7.

Jonas, S. and Rosenberg, S.N. (1986) Measurement and control of the quality of health care. In: Jones, S. (ed.) *Health Care Delivery in the United States*, pp. 416–64. New York: Springer.

Klein, R. (1983) *The Politics of the National Health Service*. London: Longman.

Kimberley, J.R. (1982) Managerial innovation and health policy: theoretical perspectives and research implications. *Journal of Health Politics, Policy and Law*, **6**, 637–52.

Körner, E. (1982; 1983) *Reports 1 to 6 of the Steering Group Health Service Information*. London: Department of Health and Social Services.

Larkin, G. (1983) *Occupational Monopoly and Modern Medicine*. London: Tavistock.

Miles, R.H. (1980) *Macro Organization Behaviour*. Glenview, Illinois: Scott Foresman.

Mintzberg, H. (1982) *The Structuring of Organizations*. Englewood Cliffs, N.J.: Prentice-Hall.

Olson, M. (1982) *The Rise and Decline of Nations*. New Haven: Yale University Press.

Parry, N. and Parry, J. (1976) *The Rise of the Medical Profession*. London: Croom Helm.

Peters, T.J. and Waterman, R.H. (1982) *In Search of Excellence*. New York: Harper Row.

Pirie, M. (1988) *Privatisation*. Aldershot: Wildwood House.

Pollitt, C., Hams, S., Hunt, D. and Marnoch, G. (1988) The reluctant manager: clinicians and budgets in the NHS. *Financial Accountability and Management*, Vol. 4 Pt. III, p. 213–33.

Powell, J.E. (1966) *A New Look at Medicine and Politics*. London: Pitman.

Pulse (1990) Comments on British Medical Association statements, April through June. Vol. 15.

Reiser, S.J. (1978) *Medicine and the Reign of Technology*. Cambridge: Cambridge University Press.

Rogers, E.M. (1983) *Diffusion of Innovations*. New York: Free Press.

Salvage, J. (1985) *The Politics of Nursing*. London: Heinemann.

Stocking, B. (1985) *Initiative and Inertia. Case Studies in the NHS*. London: Nuffield Provincial Hospitals Trust.

Strauss, A., Schatzman, L., Ehrlich, D., Bucher, R. and Sabshin, M. (1963) The hospital and its negotiated order. In: Freidson, E. (ed.) *The Hospital in Modern Society*. New York: Free Press.

Wrapp, H.E. (1967) Good managers don't make policy decisions, *Harvard Business Review*, September–October. Reprinted in J.B. Quinn, H. Mintzberg and R.M. Janes (eds) *The Strategy Process*, 1988. Englewood Cliffs, N.J.: Prentice-Hall.

2 | Crisis and Opportunity in Health Service Management

David Cox

Introduction

Discussions about the health service are often couched in highly moralistic terms – and rightly so. Caring for people who are sick and dependent, preventing ill health and suffering, providing support for people with disabilities, seeking cures for ailments and disease are all activities which relate to social concepts of virtue and ethical conduct. Incorporated into the systematic provision of welfare and health care, these moral commitments are expressed in terms of professional ethics and codes of conduct and in support for initially charitable and then state-supported hospitals and health services. At present in the UK, they help underwrite the continued popularity of the NHS so that even a government committed to radical restructuring of state welfare requires its publicity machine to affirm that the 'NHS is safe in our hands'.

The object of this chapter is to explore the nature of the moral and ethical debate that has been engendered by the introduction of general managers into the NHS. Is the NHS safe in *their* hands? Does general management have a role in establishing 'humane and egalitarian' as well as 'effective and efficient'[1] services? The purpose is normative; an enquiry into the values that may underpin management action in health care. It reviews some of the relevant literature that has emerged since the Griffiths Report and compares the debate about post-Griffiths management with some more general explorations of the role of modern management.

The argument that will be advanced links the prevalent climate of crisis in public *services* with a parallel crisis in the notion of the *public* as consumers or citizens. There is a powerful resonance in assertions that contrast the benefits of being a consumer in a free market with the dependence and subordination implied by being a client, patient, tenant, or pupil in a professionally dominated and often patronizing, sexist and racially biased public service.[2] Public services will lose their way and become the undefended victims of new right market dogma unless they are grounded in a radical reaffirmation of citizenship and the rights and obligations of the public.[3]

The critical reaction given to managerialism in the health service has raised some key dilemmas about how a managerial ethic might be grounded and relate to values and essentially political objectives. The general managers are faced with the need to challenge professional autonomy and authority and respond to consumer viewpoints and expectations. They have to do so while conforming to centrally imposed budgetary limitations, bureaucratically enforced regulations and local health authorities' wishes. It will be argued that their role provides opportunities to identify new legitimating values for the NHS and to rebuild its organizational culture.

Although critics of Griffiths, especially in the professions, highlight the new managerialism as part of the crisis in health care, it will be argued that general management does generate its own imperatives to reaffirm the core legitimating values of the health service. The underlying thesis of this Chapter is that the clients and staff of the health and care services deserve good committed general management, and it will be suggested that Griffiths may have provided an opportunity to develop this.

Bendix (1956), in his classic work on authority in industry, addresses the legitimation crisis of the first generation of professional industrial managers who were no longer the owners of early capitalist companies. The emergence of general management in the health service raises similar issues of legitimacy. The general managers need not be experts in medical care and are no longer expected to merely administer. How can they justify and legitimate their increased powers? These issues will be explored firstly at the level of the first Griffiths Report, its reception and implementation and secondly by reference to a debate about contemporary managerialism initiated by the moral philosopher Alasdair MacIntyre.

The Griffiths Report

The origins of the role of NHS general managers at Regional, District and Unit level lie in the report of the NHS Management Inquiry led by Roy (now Lord) Griffiths and published in the autumn of 1983. Previous re-organizations in 1974 and 1982 had explicitly rejected such a role. The arguments of the NHS professionals that teams of different professions were needed to make consensus decisions at each level in the NHS structure were finally and fatally challenged in Griffiths' programme for action.

General managers cannot easily appeal to many of the traditions of the

NHS to legitimate their authority. They were imposed by an 'outsider' drawing on commercial experience and explicitly rejecting many of the cherished assumptions about the uniqueness of the health services. They were to be appointed 'regardless of discipline' into a service that had revered professionalism and specialization. In some instances they were attracted from outside the health service with the explicit intention of bringing in new managerial skills and values. Above all they were introduced by a government convinced of the need to intervene in the NHS and determined to increase efficiency and contain costs (Davies, 1987; Harrison, 1988).

What resources did the first Griffiths Report offer to the new general managers seeking guidance and justification for their role and function? There is not a lot expressed in a rhetoric that might be expected to appeal to many of the predominantly professionally orientated reference groups within the NHS. Griffiths' managerialism is portrayed as a simple no-nonsense affair. The recurring themes are 'management action', 'effectiveness', 'accountability', 'performance', 'decision making', 'driving force', 'responsibility', 'devolution', 'leadership', 'initiative, urgency and vitality', 'thrust commitment and energy' and 'new style'. Apart from these evocative exhortations the cultural change was to flow from the simple appointment of general managers at each level of decision-making and responsibility. Action, in contrast to the delays and vetoes of excessive consultation and consensus, is seen as the prime value to be brought to running the NHS by general management.

Four other aspects are featured strongly. Firstly there is the requirement for more accurate costing information from management budgeting. There is an imperative to involve clinicians (i.e. hospital doctors) in management decisions and responsibility. There is a new approach to management of personnel which would reward initiative and good performance and ultimately sanction poor performance with dismissal. Finally, there is the 'underlying' commitment to 'secure the best possible services for the patient'. It is this latter legitimatory theme to which this Chapter will return.

Most of the report was concerned with 'who is in charge' and a commitment to action, with budgetary information being the main specific technical component to be contributed from commercial management practice. It was strong mindedness and getting things done that were emphasized, not professional managerial expertise or training.

Spybey (1984) schematically contrasts two rationales for contemporary industrial management: traditional and rational. Traditional management is tied to experience in, and knowledge of, one industry and its traditions. Modern rational management, a product of mergers, takeovers and conglomerates, rationalizes its activities in terms of transferable techniques and skills together with financial and personnel controls and criteria. Griffiths is clearly in the latter mould, contrasting the traditional consensus management of the health sector with modern standard commercial practice and like Spybey emphasizing the importance of rational accounting techniques as tools for cost reduction and decision-making.

The main contribution of management for Griffiths, however, is to ensure 'management action' and to bring into the health service the final authority and responsibility of management, admittedly while still wishing to preserve the best aspects of the consensus system (Griffiths Report, 1983, p. 17). This links with Storey's (1983) account of the reassertion in contemporary industrial and commercial management of the 'managerial prerogative'. This is the product of a changing economic and political environment and a new balance of power between workers and management. It is essentially an emphasis on managerial power. Action is in part about obedience, the power to force through decisions even when unpopular and the ability to make savings, changes and investments for which managers may be accountable upwards to their employers but not downwards to employee interest groups.

The professional reaction to Griffiths

It is not surprising that the reaction to Griffiths from the established NHS professions was cautious and predominantly negative. Power was being taken from and a new authority imposed on a well established and entrenched pattern of vested interests: 'Whilst such appointments may be necessary and desirable in trade and commerce they can have no place in the health service which depends upon a number of caring professions working together as a team in the interests of patients' wrote Mr Anthony Grabham, Chairman of the BMA Council in a letter to Mr Norman Fowler, then Social Services Secretary (quoted in *The Guardian*, 12 January 1984).

The Griffiths Report is respectful of medical power and seeks to involve consultants in the management process. The profession as a whole reserved its position on Griffiths and sought to preserve the established independence of the medical advisory committees and regional contracts for consultants. According to the *British Medical Journal* (10 December 1983) the Central Committee for Hospital Medical Services wanted an 'appeals mechanism against managers' decisions' and the profession to maintain its access to the Secretary of State, etc.

First reactions from the nursing profession were also critical. The Association of Nursing Administrators was quoted as saying to Norman Fowler on the publication of the report: 'The imposition of an industrial model of accountability on a service concerned with patient/client care is a cause for deep concern' (quoted in *The Guardian*, 12 January 1984). It was their members, rather than ward-level nurses, who had most to lose if the well-established Salmon levels of professional 'nursing management' were to be challenged by the introduction of general management and the relegation of what Griffiths refers to as 'functional' management.

As the appointments of general managers at regional, district and unit levels began to unfold in 1985–6 the nurse managers found that they were not getting general manager jobs in any number (Petchey, 1986, pp. 97–8). In January and February 1986 an expensive RCN advertising campaign in the press tried to reassert the need for professional management hierarchies for nurses and disparaged the appropriateness of general management. 'An ageing accountant with the clip board does not know his coccyx from his humerus' was one caricature! Traditional nursing management (one advert featured a matron) was fighting back, much too late, against the new breed of managerialists. The line taken by the RCN and in part accepted by the then DHSS and incorporated in 'guidance' to regions and districts, was that nursing was to have its professional right to offer nursing advice protected and there were to be limits to the extent to which non-nurses might enjoy managerial power over nursing staff. In many authorities a notional separation between 'professional' and 'managerial' authority was built into the new management structures as a gesture towards nursing professionalism and the sheer lobbying powers of this numerically dominant and functionally managed work group.

For both major professions in the health service the view was strongly stated that doctors and nurses *cared* for patients and had a professional role and responsibility. By implication, managers and administrators would only be concerned with 'industrial style management with all the associated ideas of productivity, efficiency and the consequent financial restraints' (Salvage, 1985, p. 158).

The New Right and public service management

The introduction of general management into the NHS has come in the context of a radical set of government policies which in turn incorporate a collage of right-wing political philosophies. Thatcherism was influenced by the ideologies and analyses of monetarism, free-market economics and political liberalism. This approach was explicitly opposed to the socialist politics under which the NHS and the welfare state were established in the post-War period and to the 'consensus' politics under which they have survived. Griffiths can be seen as part of the desire to deregulate professions, control public expenditure, introduce market discipline and commercial and industrial models of management. Expenditure controls, Rayner scrutinies, privatization, competitive tendering and a willingness to challenge the power of both trade unions and the professions were a consistent feature of Conservative government in the 1980s.

To what extent did this pattern of 'New Right' thinking offer a positive role for public service management and a basis for legitimating the new general managers? By implication, management in the public services was suspect from this ideological stand-point. The expansion of public services

was seen as being in part driven by the ambitions of those professionals
and administrators whose careers and prospects derived from that expansion, the Niskanen (1971) effect.

Some of the Griffiths Report implies this critique. Private-sector management is more concerned with cost control, effectiveness, speed of
decision-making and the quality of the service to the customer. Competition is the spur to good management and there was an expectation that
many of the new general managers would be attracted in from industry
and bring in appropriate standards and techniques. Short-term contracts,
higher than Whitley salaries, and performance-related pay would guarantee
results because of managers' self-interest.

General managers cannot find a very secure base for legitimating their
activities in the intellectual tradition that motivates their progenitors.
While controlling costs, setting targets, ensuring action and making
decisions are all important activities the implication is that they are all
done much better in the private sector anyway. There is little incentive
to be offering a vision of the future health service in the context of a
government which is profoundly suspicious of service values and looking at new ways of diversifying health care provision (Davies, 1987).
Paradoxically, at a time when management theorists and trainers have
been emphasizing the importance of 'culture'[4] and the value-driven nature
of management activity in either the private or public sectors, the
Thatcher Government's attacks on the public-sector employees in general
have served to undermine morale and a moral basis for leadership.

The Thatcher government's approach to the management of the public
services should not necessarily be seen as a coherent whole. Like most
initiatives in government, it was a bricolage of partially conflicting elements derived from different ideologies and pressures. Two underlying
sets of ideas and prejudices regarding the management of services can be
deciphered.

Firstly, there was the managerialism of big business, of oligopoly and
the large corporation. Big capital, especially in the form of Mrs Thatcher's
favourite retail chains, Sainsbury's (as represented by Griffiths) and Marks
& Spencer (as represented by Rayner), provides one model of private
business. Here the emphasis is on speed of decision-making, coordination,
accountability, setting and reviewing objectives, good financial controls
and information, cost improvement, consumer loyalty and public image
and responsiveness.

Secondly, however, there was the ideological influence of *laissez-faire*
and the New Right. Here the model is small business – the entrepreneur in
the competitive marketplace – whose main enemy may well be the large
corporation as much as taxing governments. From these roots comes the
emphasis on market criteria, prices (not costs), competition, tendering,
privatization and the casualization of manual and managerial labour. From
this perspective the NHS is not just a large corporation needing better
management but the symbol of 'socialism', dependency, professional self-

indulgence and the undermining of a competitive economy. This, in part, explains the willingness to encourage private medicine, 'internal markets', competitive tendering (see Ascher, 1987) and more recently, hospitals 'opting out' which serve to undermine the comprehensive nature of the NHS even when policy analysts have long documented the way the NHS serves to contain overall health costs in comparison to other western countries.

The clash of big and small business values in government policies comes out particularly in the drive to open out cleaning and other contracts to competitive tendering. This has become mandatory for political rather than economic reasons. As Cousins' interviews show, many managers would rather award contracts to their own workers and retain a higher degree of control over costs and the quality of service (Cousins, 1987, p. 174). Political interference in the logic of managing and developing a large service organization is suggested to be the main reason that the first Chairman of the Management Board, Victor Paige, resigned (see Cousins, 1987, p. 170).

The authoritarian and centralist aspects of Thatcherism have been commented on (Stacey, 1988) by political critics who point to the contradictions of a

> Government which, while professing liberal values of free competition and private enterprise, has strengthened central government control in many aspects of life in a manner unprecedented in Britain. . . .

Stacey sees the attacks on the autonomy of the professions as part of the process of taming and weakening all those structures with political power and resources sufficient to oppose or obstruct government programmes (Stacey, 1988, p. 14).

But this centralism while seeming to weaken the independence of health authorities and professions also affects general management. Within a managerialist framework, if general managers are to be merely the agents of central Whitehall control, as their critics suspect (e.g. Cousins, 1987; Widgery, 1988), then they will not enjoy the delegated autonomy to manage promised by Griffiths. Similarly, if the current NHS reform further exposes their performance to nationally determined measures of output priorities then the new health service managers will not have the alternative of accountability to a locally mediated policy framework.

The socialist critique of general management

For both the Left and the Right in UK politics, the NHS is often taken as a symbol of socialism in practice. Many critiques from the Left have focussed on the power of the medical profession, ever since Bevan struck a deal with them in 1948 to determine the conditions under which health care is provided. This approach is essentially pluralist in its analysis, the 1945 settlement being a victory for working-class pressure but the subsequent shaping of the NHS being determined by medical hegemony. More recently as Marxist and feminist ideas have begun to influence critical social analysis, then the NHS has been viewed more sceptically as part of the social reproduction of labour power and ultimately shaped by the requirements of the capitalist mode of production (Navarro, 1976).

The Labour Party's response to Griffiths was equivocal. In part it was seen as an attack on both the professions and the health service unions, a cover up for the inadequate funding of the service and a means of facilitating cuts. Moreover, general management was a further move towards centralization from the then DHSS and the lessening of democratic influences from parliament or health authorities and, like competitive tendering, the extension of commercial values into public service. However, it became clear that general managers would have been retained if Labour had won the election in 1987, alongside elected health authorities. This was partly on the grudging grounds that the NHS could not stand another reorganization but also the suggestion that managers could be targeted on different policy objectives.[5]

Two recent accounts of the current health service from left-wing perspectives are very critical of Griffiths and hold little promise of legitimating a conscientious role for general management. Widgery (1988) sees general managers as essentially obedient to increasingly centralized control, most were 'merely' promoted administrators, and he (like the BMA) rejects the parallels with business management as 'nonsense' because 'there is not, or ought not to be, a profit motive in the provision of health' (Widgery, 1988, pp. 43–4).

Cousins (1987) provides a much more analytic sociology of state welfare work and organization based in the thriving 'labour process' tradition of industrial sociology. One chapter based on field work in south-east England looks at the NHS as an example of the restructuring of welfare work and focusses on general management and the contracting out of ancillary services.

Cousins and her respondents (professionals and trade unionists in two health authorities) offer a very negative evaluation of the initial impact of general management. Managers are appointed on short-term contracts to enforce central control and close hospital wards and beds (Cousins, 1987, p. 165):

> Evidence from the authors' study suggested that there was a tendency for managers to treat the health service as a set of commodities, of plant, equipment, and manpower, which they had the right to manage as they saw fit rather than as being held in trust for the public.

Cousins is sensitive to the legitimatory problems faced by general managers as they become exposed to the political pressures from professionals, unions and community health groups. Her overall assessment is very negative as shown by the following quotation (Cousins, 1987, p. 171):

> However, the new managerialism has caused considerable disruption, lowering morale and the moral commitment of staff, undermining the effectiveness of patient care, and exacerbating the tensions between managerial values and the 'collaborative' or caring values orientated to the health needs of the population.

By implication, perhaps the existing patterns of NHS organization, medically dominated consensus management and the functional hierarchies of nursing management are to be preferred to the new arrangements. The balance of local interests helped to protect services from change and cut-backs and nursing management had provided greater career opportunities for women than the new general management structure (Cousins, 1987, p. 167).

Finally, Cousins suggests that attempts by general managers to legitimate and defend their role will be counter productive to the service (Cousins, 1987, p. 169):

> To the extent that general managers can convince the public and employees, by their use of language, that their practices are in the public interest then their scope for further reductions in service and more coercive controls of the labour process are possible ... .

Petchey (1986) has a more dialectical assessment of the same pressures and contradictions. In introducing general management, the Government has made the financial rationing of services much more obvious to the public and a direct line of accountability has been created, 'a line that leads direct to the door of the Secretary of State'. Policies and their effects are less likely to be fudged behind a complex of committees and interprofessional negotiations. Secondly, Petchey sees Griffiths as being a 'challenge to forty years of professional domination of the NHS' (Petchey, 1986, p. 101):

> It is clear that the medical profession itself has to be controlled, and if Griffiths should achieve this, then strangely enough it may turn out that his impact will not be entirely regressive.

Management after virtue

In the NHS, as in other public services, traditional administrative and professional frames of meaning can be contrasted with the new managerialist ideologies. This section steps back from the immediate debates about Griffiths to examine some recent thinking about the contemporary role of management in general.

MacIntyre (1981) reiterates the proposition that modern societies have no concept of virtue, of what it is to lead the good life nor to die a good death. This is because they are not communities subscribing to common sets of values on which an ethics of conduct could be based. There is no moral basis for action and moralists pursue fictions left over from more certain times while rival groups protest and make incommensurable claims to rights, utility or justice. Philosophers can give us only 'emotivism'; value is the arbitrary assertion of preference and desire.

MacIntyre's treatise on moral philosophy is unusual in that within it he develops an extended critique of modern management. He claims that while aspiring to be effective in scientifically manipulating people to achieve goals, modern management has no criteria for evaluating those goals. Furthermore, transferable management 'skills' are not based, he claims, in any genuine scientific expertise and he is scathing about the pretensions of management science to predict and control the social world. Managerialism for MacIntyre is the nihilistic triumph of will and power in achieving objectives and getting things done. The success of the bureaucratic manager is based in the shallow manipulative success of boardroom histrionics (MacIntyre, 1981, p. 102) not in the integrity of any values or goals served nor in any genuine scientifically based training and skill. The claims made by Griffiths for general management in the NHS may be seen to epitomize this critique. Management skills developed in the commercial sector are held to be equally applicable in the world of health care. Many of the early professional reactions outlined above reflect a distaste for the intrusion of business managerialism into the sacrosanct ethical world of professional and caring values.

MacIntyre's insight into the 'histrionic' aspect of modern management is interesting. Cousins refers to the success, or otherwise, of the general managers 'use of language' (Cousins 1987, p. 189) while the 'culture of excellence' literature highlights the myths and stories told about successful managers (Peters and Waterman, 1982). Strong and Robinson's (1988, p. 54) fascinating recent ethnography of the introduction of general management in a sample of district health authorities contains examples of the heady and 'inspirational' meetings they attended. Similarly, there are dramatic descriptions of the new managers in action confronting especially the entrenched medical profession. In the author's research, general managers have emphasized in interviews and displayed in observations an ability to show passionate concern for the values of care. Elaborating management values was an important element in the early days of general management in the NHS.

There are problems with MacIntyre's argument. It is doubtful if many practising managers cite social science as their legitimating ideology. Effectiveness perhaps, but based in action, leadership and tough minded-ness rather than in theory, with the partial exception, as in Griffiths, of management accounting. Research on what managers do, rather than what they are taught on courses, emphasizes the unscheduled reactive 'bittiness' of managerial work rather than the systematic implementation of plans (Mintzberg, 1975).

However, MacIntyre's critique is powerful. Few people, including those in private or public service management, like to be thought of as less than at least potentially 'virtuous'. One management writer who has taken MacIntyre's argument seriously is Anthony (1986) in a critique of the education and performance of UK management. His thesis is that modern UK management has retreated into concern for professionalized 'technique' and purely economic objectives. In doing so it has neglected management's fundamental 'governmental' function, the responsibility for the control and direction of labour. Anthony has sensed the legitimation problems attendant on the revival of the managerial prerogative indicated by Storey (1983).

Anthony develops a view of organizations as moral communities in themselves, in part held together by informal relationships. Managers' 'histrionics' or story telling is not a disguise but their real activity. Managers then have a 'narrative' role in shaping and holding together the social organizations that they govern. For Anthony

> the foundation of managerial authority, its legitimation by those subordinate to it, cannot be assured by other means than the acceptance by management of its responsibility to the general community and for the government of its own.

And (Anthony, 1986, p. 198):

> The authority of management must rest upon a moral base, secure in a concern for the integrity and the good of the community that it governs.

The legitimacy of general management has been widely challenged and its origins in the Griffiths Report and the political context in which it has been introduced into the NHS do not go very far to resolve the dilemma of the conscientious general manager. Anthony's book is a courageous and creative attempt to think through MacIntyre's powerful and damning critique of *all* modern management and to develop a legitimate conceptual and moral base for the realities of management practice.

There is an interesting contradiction within the contemporary Western approach to management which is picked up by Cousins and by Abercrombie *et al.* (1986). They both point to the paradox that while Western capitalist ideology encourages possessive, competitive individualism, the more successful capitalist economy of Japan appears to benefit competitively from the collectivism that underpins its large corporations. Abercrombie *et al.* contrast 'consensus' management in Japan and the sort of Western corporate management practices implied to some extent in the Griffiths Report and further exaggerated by the *laissez-faire* ideologies of the enterprise culture. They cite (Ouchi, 1981, quoted in Abercrombie *et al.*, 1986, p. 127) a specification of Japanese management that could as easily be a characterization of traditional NHS management arrangements!

At the management level, group decision-making processes depend on consultation and consensus among peers and on collective responsibility, which ensures that no individual manager is associated with a particular decision.

Abercrombie *et al.* continue (p. 127):

These processes are clearly alien to western management practices that demand individual initiative and responsibility, and to a culture that sanctions the pursuit of policies that are unpopular elsewhere within the organisation, provided that they can be presented as technically correct (for example, the endorsement of 'macho' managers who demonstrate their individual strength of will by taking 'tough' decisions against opposition).

For Anthony, all organizations including the NHS, are collective entities, moral communities. Managements have to take responsibility for leading these communities. In this, UK commercial and industrial management, especially in the form celebrated in the 'enterprise culture', may have something to learn from their Japanese counterparts and even the NHS.

Consumers and citizens

Anthony (1986, p. 198) asserts that management has a governmental role and that in part this must involve acceptance of a responsibility to the general community. How might this responsibility to the general community be exercised in the general management of the NHS? Can there be a measure of consensus in a national health service as to the public good to be pursued? The NHS management's responsibility to the general community must turn on normative judgements about the role of public services and indeed what is meant by 'public'. Much of the writing and discussion about the health service and general management does accept or imply a moral discourse about public service, about quality, consumer satisfaction, efficient use of resources and 'care'.

Griffiths (DHSS, 1983, p. 10) draws an unfavourable comparison between attitudes of the traditional NHS and the private sector where,

Businessmen have a keen sense of how well they are looking after their customers. Whether the NHS is meeting the needs of the patient, and the community, and can prove that it is doing so is open to question.

The Report (p. 10) quotes a government statement from 1944.

the real need is to bring the country's full resources to bear upon reducing ill-health and promoting good health in all its citizens.

Later on, the Report states (p. 11) that

as a caring, quality service, the NHS has to balance the interests of the patient, the community, the tax-payer and the employees.

These issues of public service, of balancing interests can be related to notions of a civic culture and the rights and duties of citizenship. In the UK it is a concept that has never been well established or defined legally and yet was widely used during the post-War phase of social reconstruction which saw the foundation of the NHS. Marshall (1963) chronicles what he saw as the steady evolution of citizenship from civil, to political, to social rights. The welfare state was another step forward guaranteeing adequate standards of subsistence, shelter, education and health to all citizens and offering protection from the harmful effects of the free market. In the post-War settlement, the entitlements of citizens provided the legitimation for a public health service which was free at the point of use and sought to give equal treatment to all citizens on a basis of need.[6]

Such a concept of citizenship promising a consensus on which the legitimation of public services might be based seems to have lost some of its popularity and effectiveness over the next 40 years. In the context of post-Griffiths health care, the consumer has replaced the citizen. Consumer satisfaction may be seen to have more of a cutting edge than citizenship rights. The citizen wanted publicly accountable services freed from the fear of commercial exploitation and protection from the sub-standard products of unregulated markets. The modern consumer is seen to want services which are prompt, competitive, respond to researched demands, offer choice and ensure satisfaction.

Marshall's account of the slow march towards full democracy has been taken up by Turner in *Citizenship and Capitalism* (1986). He shows how the advance of citizenship rights, civil, political and social, was the outcome of political struggles by successive emerging political groups. The propertied male middle class, the male working class, women, black people and ethnic minorities, and more recently gay men and lesbians, have campaigned for citizenship rights. These rights are not in any way guaranteed and gains made can be lost in political reaction as evidenced by retreats on equal opportunities policies or attacks like Clause 29.

Pluralistic claims to rights and services are fought for, but against a weakening consensus and no legal guarantees of the civil, political or social rights of all citizens. In a perceptive discussion, Ferris (1985) claims that the problems of the Keynesian welfare state are not just economic; they also result from a failure of moral vision. The institutions of the post-War period and the benefits they provided (social security, housing, education and health care), were only an arena for the instrumental politics of distribution. They were not underpinned by 'war socialism' or the 'solidarity of working class struggle' and no strongly felt consensus about shared values or mutual dependency emerged to consolidate feelings and obligation of reciprocity. Expectations of many services declined and they became the stigmatized marginal provision of a dual society. This was clear in the case of social security and has become so in housing. In the late 1980s, the education and health services have become the terrain in which the choice between universal state services and a mixed economy of welfare implying dual citizenship is being addressed.

Ferris' assessment of the decline of a consensus basis for citizenship is summed up thus (Ferris, 1985, p. 64):

> for any political group once its collective distributive claims are met, public life simply becomes an irksome burden to be left to salaried functionaries.

He believes that

> a broader view of citizenship is needed to secure the rights and freedom of those groups who are to varying degrees excluded from full participation in social and political life.

Others have developed critiques of the way the public health and welfare services have failed to enhance the citizenship of consumers over the last 40 years. Critics from both Left and Right suggest that services have been driven by 'producer' values and provided in a centralized, paternalistic, bureaucratic and professional manner. From these perspectives, the vested interests of the professions and public service unions are overriding consumer interests. In local government, Hoggert and Hambleton (1987) suggest that policies for privatization and decentralization are different political responses to frustration with the experience of 30 or more years of paternalistic bureaucracy which left the local administrations with few active supporters.

In a recent Fabian pamphlet, Corrigan *et al.* (1988) write of the crisis in public service and reiterate the claim that the welfare bureaucracies have 'taken upon themselves to designate what the public needs rather than responding to its demands' and 'They see the public as a passive receiver of services rather than as citizens who have obligations to and rights over institutions' (p. 10). As Corrigan sees it (p. 12), the relationship between the welfare services and the public 'had no real possibilities of reciprocity'.

Seeing the health service as responding to consumers or customers is one of the features of the Griffiths Report. How does such a concept relate to more traditional characterizations of the recipients of public health care?

Patients have conditions and problems that medical care seeks to cure; they may have other needs as well such as dignity but the concept specifies a degree of passivity. Protection of their interests is largely left to the ethical codes of self-regulating professionals and complaints procedures. 'Client' as a term originated in the independent patron who hires the specialist professional to perform a service. In the post-War period, it has tended to be devalued to refer to the beneficiary of a state directed 'intervention'. Both terms now have connotations of passivity, gratitude and relative powerlessness.

The notion of the consumer or the customer is associated with the new managerialism but is this any more empowering? Stacey (1976) claims that the health-service consumer is a misconception. We all play an active role in maintaining or producing our own health; health care cannot be consumed like any other product or service on the market. This view can, however, be countered by the argument that the same is true of much consumption in the private marketplace. Food has to be cooked and prepared, cars maintained and driven, clothes worn, cleaned and assembled into a 'look', holidays actively enjoyed (!) and much furniture has to be built up at home from flat packs (Huws, 1988).

The power of the individual consumer is seen to come from the free market with the ability to make an informed choice and switch preferences to another supplier. For advocates of the free market, the objection to state services is that they are often a monopoly and their power is not limited by freedom of choice and alternatives. Consumerism may be seen as challenging the traditional paternalism of public services. However, even without the reality of a free market and sufficient income for all to make choices, consumerism has come to be associated with listening to customers, assessing the quality of a service and overcoming the 'organisational indifference' (Hall, 1974) of mass public services.

'Consumerism' as a collective movement represented by the Consumers Association in the UK and Ralph Nader in the USA is about organizing the countervailing power of consumers to challenge corporate power through information, testing and legal action. In this sense it is a reflection of imperfection in the market economy and the need for negotiation of preferences and protection through pressure group activity. Public service managers share with their commercial counterparts the threat of negative publicity and a loss of public support. Community Health Council representations, individual complaints, litigation and campaigns about waiting lists and cancelled operations do reflect a form of consumer power. Paradoxically, as in the case of the Birmingham Children's Hospital heart operations which became material for parliamentary questions, such campaigns may reinforce existing biases in the pattern of health care towards high-technology acute medicine.

Jones and Jowell (1987) welcome consumerism as a new form in social policy supported by a seeming political consensus of the Left and the Right. They caution (p. 19)

> too close an analogy with the market place because personal social services' development is not based on a model of consumer driven market forces but on a complex combination of political mandate, professional judgement and statutory requirements.

Nevertheless, seeing clients and carers as consumers they suggest (p. 19) enables managers and policy-makers to question the

> large organisations whose systems for service delivery are often blatantly unsympathetic and indifferent to the human sensitivities of our clients.

Their suggestions in the article and in the activities of the Community Care Special Action Project in Birmingham really revolve around issues of humanity, individuality and consultation. Jones and Jowell describe the programme of informal consultations with carers, not 'representatives', conducted through the Action Project and the way this forces managers to look at their services in a new light.

The power of citizenship as a validating value for public services is that it seeks to establish the rights and services that all members of a society are entitled to enjoy. It is an inherently reciprocal concept, producers, managers, consumers and carers are all citizens irrespective of wealth, gender, ethnicity or race. Citizenship invokes the mutual obligations that sustain a society. It must also involve needs, wants and choices, but the choices are at the policy level as well as the individual. This must imply some form of democratic participation in health authorities which determine local policy for management action. In that context responsiveness to the citizen as consumer could follow. Enhancing citizenship would provide a context in which public services and their managements could be developed and given a new vision and purpose.

Managers in the public services, including the NHS, have a choice. They can identify their services with the enhancement of citizenship and a respect for consumers' rights and humanity. The alternative is to become the supervisors of the institutions of a new Poor Law offering a stigmatized second-class service to second-class citizenry who will never be recognized as 'people like themselves'. A wholesale revalorization of the public services requires a radical review of citizenship rights and obligations but this has become an important element of contemporary political debate.

There are, however, signs that a desire for self-respect amongst health service managers themselves leads them into a consideration of the underlying values that drive their services and sustain the positive aspects of the organizational cultures within which they work. For example, Solihull Health Authority recently had the courage to publish the results of an 'away day' for members and senior officers. This was an agreement on 'a set of very basic values that would guide our management philosophy'. Value 1 was 'Treat others as you would expect to be treated' with the aim 'to recognise the individuality and independence of people' (Jackson, 1986).

Conclusion

The introduction of general management into the NHS can be assessed as a challenge to a medical domination which has to some extent protected it from governmental interference. In the service of recent governments, managers have been working under a deluge of central directives[7] and recent indications of determination to remove local authority representatives from health authorities and let hospitals 'opt out'. However, in a different political context, their efforts could be directed in the service of different policies. Furthermore, there are elements in the role of general management itself which encourage an identification with the service and the consumer. Linking the values of the service to a revitalized notion of citizenship and providing more local democratic participation in health authorities rather than less would provide a radically different context for the implementation of health policy.

Management is needed in the health service as in other public services. It is needed to develop services just as much as to cut them. It is naive of critics on the Left to assume that good quality complex services can be supplied effectively without a managerial role being performed well. Getting things done including responding to complaints or making progress on equal opportunities will require the managerial drive celebrated by Griffiths. Critics of the NHS from the Right with their enthusiasm for market forces, entrepreneurship and competition miss the importance of management and organizational values in any large modern service organization whether privately or publicly owned.

A retreat to the medically dominated consensus of professions as an overt way of running the health service is unlikely to service the needs of the citizen consumer nor the ambitions of governments seeking to achieve policy objectives and contain costs. Management has to be general, responsible for a whole product or service and for the division of labour that produces it. Coordination and accountability are the core of the management role, responsibility for setting goals, bringing together resources and people, monitoring and evaluating performance and a keen sense of the service to the customer can only be carried out on a generalist basis. The answer to the RCN's advertising campaign of 1986 lies in the general management potential of the nurse role, not in reviving long functional hierarchies.

Cousins (1987) sees the political environment as a limit to general management. However, balancing internal and external political pressures is a key element in the general management role in the NHS as in any other organization or industry. Mobilizing support, defending services and looking for opportunities to conserve and redirect resources, for example from institutional to community care, requires managerial skill, expertise and commitment. There is a need to assert a role for general management in the public services which is more sophisticated than either the crude, industrial entrepreneurial model celebrated by some newspaper tycoons or the narrow technicist models of management advocated by some business schools and consultants (Anthony, 1986; Hunter, 1988).

The empirical work of researchers Strong and Robinson (1988) shows how the imperatives facing general managers in the NHS demand that they show a vision of the service and its future that takes responsibility for 'balancing the books' but goes beyond asset stripping and makes them critical of central interference and market models. Strong and Robinson

(p. 116) indicate a high level of commitment to the values of the NHS amongst the new general managers.

There is a paradox in the 'crossover' of public and private management philosophies. The Conservative Government is keen to hold up the image of the industrial and commercial manager as a model for the hidebound bureaucratic and professionalized public services. Meanwhile some management thinkers have been holding up the NHS as a model to private-sector management. Both Burns (1981) and Anthony (1986) see the collaborative culture of the NHS as an example of the sort of common purpose and identity that any modern management should aspire to generate in their corporation.

The challenge for those who wish to see public services that are effective, efficient, humane and egalitarian is to link those values to the public support of these services. Ensuring that support requires competent management of resources, leadership of staff, a flexible and responsive service and a systematic defence of the services in face of the budgetary constraints and negative attitudes of government. To do anything like a competent management job in the NHS, the new general managers will have to become its principal defenders by gaining the support of staff and consumers, improving performance and becoming a vociferous lobby for resources. The general management movement initiated by Griffiths legitimates its activity in part by reference to quality of service and consumer satisfaction. In health care, these values cannot be grounded in the emotivism of market preferences. They have to be set in the context of the intrinsic worth of all citizens in a pluralistic society and a commitment to equity and service.

Notes

1 These four concepts are used by Robinson and Strong (1987) and in the Open University (1985) text.
2 See for example Centre for Contemporary Cultural Studies (1981), Fenton (1985), Corrigan et al. (1988), McNaught (1988), Roberts (1985), Orr (1987).
3 New Statesman and Society has championed this debate through 1988 leading up to the Charter 88 Campaign. See also Marquand (1988), Ferris (1985), Plant (1988).
4 Peters and Waterman (1982), Hunter (1988).
5 See commentary in Health Service Journal, 6 October 1988, p. 1151, 'New Realism and the NHS'.
6 Turner (1986, p. 7) in a very useful review of the relationship quotes Rose et al. (1984, p. 152): 'Citizenship hinders the carrying through of market principles; for example, a citizen has a right to health care regardless of any ability to pay.'
7 See Strong and Robinson (1988) and evidence of both Institute of Health Service Management and National Association of Health Authorities to Parliamentary Select Committee on Social Services quoted in Health Service Journal, 4 June 1987.

References

Abercrombie, N., Hill, S. and Turner, B.S. (1986) *Sovereign Individuals of Capitalism*. London: Allen & Unwin.
Anthony, P.D. (1986) *The Foundation of Management*. London: Tavistock.
Ascher, K. (1987) *The Politics of Privatisation: The Contracting Out of Public Services*. London: Macmillan.
Bendix, R. (1956) *Work and Authority in Industry*. New York: John Wiley.
Burns, T. (1981) A Comparative Study of the Administrative Structure and Organisational Processes in Selected Areas in the NHS. London: SSRC Research Report.
Centre for Contemporary Cultural Studies (1981) *Unpopular Education: Schooling and Social Democracy in England Since 1944*. London: Hutchinson.
Corrigan, P., Jones, T., Lloyd, J. and Young, J. (1988) Socialism, merit and efficiency. *Fabian Society Pamphlet*, No. 530. London: Fabian Society.
Cousins, C. (1987) *Controlling Social Welfare: A Sociology of State Welfare Work and Organisation*. Brighton: Wheatsheaf.
Davies, C. (1987) Viewpoint. Things to come: the NHS in the next decade. *Sociology of Health and Illness*, **9**(3), 303–17.
Department of Health and Social Security (1983) *NHS Management Inquiry (The Griffiths Report)*. London: DHSS.
Fenton, S. (1985) *Race, Health and Welfare*: Bristol: University of Bristol.
Ferris, J. (1985) Citizenship and the crisis of the welfare state. In: Bean, P., Ferris, J. and Whynes, D. (eds) *In Defence of Welfare*. London: Tavistock.
Hall, A. (1974) *The Point of Entry: A Study of Client Reception in the Social Services*. London: Allen & Unwin.
Harrison, S. (1988) The workforce and the new managerialism. In: Maxwell, R. (ed.) *Reshaping the National Health Service*. Oxford: Policy Journals, Transaction Books.
Hoggert, P. and Hambleton, R. (1987) Beyond bureaucratic paternalism. In: Hoggert, P. and Hambleton, R. (eds) *Decentralisation and Democracy: Localising Public Services*. Bristol: School for Advanced Urban Studies.
Hunter, D. (1988) The impact of research on restructuring the British National Health Service. *Journal of Health Administrative Education*, **6**(3), 537–53.
Huws, U. (1988) Consuming fashions. *New Statesman and Society*, 19 August, 32–4.
Jackson, C. (1986) Values that hold the key. *Twenty Two*. Autumn. West Midlands Regional Health Authority.
Jones, A. and Jowell, T. (1987) May the force be with you. *Social Services Insight*, 10 July, 19–21.
MacIntyre, A. (1981) *After Virtue*. Notre Dame: University of Notre Dame Press.
McNaught, A. (1988) *Race and Health Policy*. Beckenham: Croom Helm.
Marquand, D. (1988) *The Unprincipled Society*. London: Fontana.
Marshall, T.H. (1963) Citizenship and social class. *Sociology at the Crossroads*, Ch. 4. London: Heinemann.
Mintzberg, H. (1975) The manager's job: folklore and fact. *Harvard Business Review*, **53**, 49–61.
Navarro, V. (1976) *Medicine Under Capitalism*. London: Croom Helm.
Niskanen, W. (1971). *Bureaucracy and Representative Government*. Chicago: Aldine.

Open University (1985) *Caring for Health: Dilemmas and Prospects*. Milton Keynes: Open University Press.

Orr, J. (ed.) (1987) *Women's Health in the Community*. Chichester: John Wiley.

Ouchi, W.G. (1981) *Theory Z*. New York: Avon.

Petchey, R. (1986) The Griffiths reorganisation of the National Health Service: Fowlerism by stealth? *Critical Social Policy*, **17**, 87–101.

Peters, T. and Waterman, R. (1982) *In Search of Excellence*. New York: Harper Row.

Plant, R. (1988) Citizenship, rights and socialism. *Fabian Society Pamphlet*, No. 531. London: Fabian Society.

Roberts, H. (1985) *Patient Patients: Women and their Doctors*. London: Pandora.

Robinson, J. and Strong, P. (1987) *Professional Nursing Advice After Griffiths: An Interim Report*. Warwick: Nursing Policy Studies Centre.

Rose, D., Vogler, C., Marshall, G. and Newby, H. (1984) Economic restructuring: The British experience. *Annals of the American Academy of Political and Social Science*, **475**, 137–57.

Salvage, J. (1985) *The Politics of Nursing*. London: Heinemann.

Spybey, T. (1984) Traditional and professional frames of meaning of management. *Sociology*, **18**(4), 550–62.

Stacey, M. (1976) The health service consumer: a sociological misconception. In: Stacey, M. (ed.) *The Sociology of the National Health Service*. Keele: Sociological Review monograph.

Stacey, M. (1988) Power, responsibility and accountability: a critical analysis of the British medical profession. *Medical Sociology News*, **14**(1), 10–39.

Storey, J. (1983) *Managerial Prerogative and the Question of Control*. London: Routledge.

Strong, P. and Robinson, J. (1988) *New Model Management: Griffiths and the NHS*. Warwick: Nursing Policy Studies Centre.

Turner, B.S. (1986) *Citizenship and Capitalism: The Debate over Reformism*. London: Allen & Unwin.

Widgery, D. (1988) *The National Health Service: A Radical Perspective*. London: Hogarth.

3 | Professionals as Gatekeepers: The Role of Doctors in the Pharmaceutical Value Chain

Mo H. Malek, Peter G. Davey and William Scott

Introduction

The general perception with regard to 'health care' is that it constitutes a unique commodity and should be treated separately outside the realm of economic analysis, or at least, in an exclusive compartment with its own specific rules, regulations and organizational behaviour. Exactly because of this perceived specificity of 'health commodity', public sectors of different countries has committed resources, to varying degrees, of course, to finance the provision of a public health service. Nowhere are these peculiarities reflected better than in the behaviour of the pharmaceutical product market. The public health administrators are caught up between two seemingly irreconcilable perceptions of what the public health should be. On the one hand, provision of publicly financed and produced goods would make strict application of conventional criteria of economic efficiency difficult, if not impossible. On the other hand, they have come under increasing pressure (especially in recent years) to improve on their performance. This is the classical problem of optimization (of efficiency) under constraints (external and internal), given a specific market structure. The purpose of this chapter is to relay the recent experience of Tayside Health Board in dealing with this problem. The first part of the chapter is a brief outline of the theoretical considerations and the second part gives an account of the organization and institutional changes taking place at the local level.

Figure 3.1 Free market model of distribution

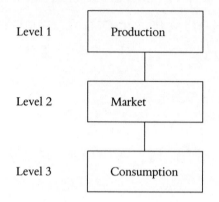

Theoretical background

As any elementary economic textbook would tell us, the process of production and price determination in any unregulated market is subject to interactions between supply and demand in a fairly straightforward manner. The producers, of whom there should be many, use the most productive technique to make the commodity. Thus produced, the commodity will be promoted to reach the consumers who have access to information and are free to exercise their sovereign rights (purchasing power) as a vote of confidence to a particular producer by buying his product. As such, all stages of production, distribution, purchasing and consumption are conducted through a market mechanism with little or no need of government intervention or interference. Ideally, allocation of resources would be optimal, the consumers would be satisfied and the least cost production of those goods and services would ensure that efficiency is maximized. In this process the market is the final arbiter in the selection of inputs, technique of production, marketing and distribution. There is natural selection of the least cost method both at the stage of production as well as the consumption of the final input. In achieving this, the market acts in a subtle manner as if the producer and the consumers meet each other face to face. Indeed the famous invisible hand of the market would ensure the equilibrium (see Fig. 3.1). In contrast, the pharmaceutical product market is rigged with restrictions and regulations at all stages from its inception (research, development and testing), to production (promotion and distribution) and finally its consumption (prescription, storage, purchase and use). Government actively intervenes to supervise and regulate the market, the consumer's 'ignorance' as opposed to consumer's sovereignty is taken to be the guiding principle and prescribers act as an additional intermediary between the producer and the consumer. As such, prescribers have

Figure 3.2 Institutionalized market for drugs

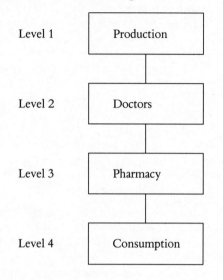

assumed an authority which supplants some of the functions expected to be performed by the market mechanism.

On the production side, the pharmaceutical industry is heavily capital-intensive and research-based with a relatively high cost of R & D giving rise to both its specific cost structure as well as affecting its long-term strategic allocation of resources over time and across different countries. Langle *et al.* (1985) estimate £40–120 million to be the average cost of introducing any new medicament into the market. The uncertainty and risk associated with the development of new drugs, in an area where the pace of technological development is fast, is frequently taken to be the main justification for existence of a wider than average profit margin. Also the high cost of R & D and the degree of capital intensity act as formidable barriers to entry, thus ensuring that the supply structure in therapeutic sub-markets remains oligopolistic with all its consequent implications for prices and output. Consequently, competition in such markets is heavily concentrated on non-price areas of research, quality, marketing and information.

Introduction of the UK National Health Service (NHS) to the demand side of the equation only increases the complexity of the problem. The simplicity of the market structure for an ordinary commodity as exemplified in Fig. 3.1 is now replaced with that of Fig. 3.2. The production and consumption ends of the market in both cases are identical and very little can be done in the latter case to improve economic efficiency in these two areas. The market as a catalyst for attaining equilibrium is now replaced by the doctors who initiate demand on behalf

of the final users and the pharmacists who are engaged in the process
of procurement and distribution. Given the irrelevancy of the external
(central) governmental budget constraints in our analysis, the search for
factors potentially responsible for loss of economic efficiency through
replacement of the market must be concentrated at these two levels (Levels
2 and 3 of Fig. 3.2). At Level 2 there are two distinct but interrelated
problems.

The first one concerns the perceived right of doctors to initiate demand
for medicines based on the principle of clinical freedom, namely, 'The
right of the doctor to do as he thinks is best for an *individual* patient'.[1]
Exercising this power raises the possible dichotomy between clinical
choice and economic efficiency. As Maynard has put it, there are three
possibilities but the two concepts of clinical and economic efficiency only
coincide in one of these three alternatives:[2]

> In the first place, a medical procedure may be clinically efficient, i.e.
> the most effective therapy available to improve the health status of an
> individual suffering from a particular complaint, regardless of cost.
> Secondly, a procedure may be cost-effective, i.e. the cheapest
> therapy available to achieve a given therapeutic end, with the value
> of outcome being unquestioned. Finally, a procedure may meet the
> criterion of economic efficiency as defined above, i.e. cost is
> minimised, outcome benefit is maximised, and the services provided
> are those most highly valued by society.

The second problem arises from the fact that despite the total
commitment for putting the patients first and adherence to the principle of
clinical freedom, there is surprisingly little scientific evaluation of clinical
efficacy and performance of drugs in relation to cost. Furthermore, the
NHS philosophy of universal provision of health care (among them drugs)
implies that neither the physicians who prescribe the drugs nor the patients
who are the final consumers have any interest and/or incentive in cost
minimization. As such the price elasticity of demand for medicament for
both groups is zero or close to zero (allowing for prescription charges).
However, this is not a problem exclusive to the NHS. In any social
institution whether public (like the NHS) or private (like insurance companies in the USA) in which the consumers are not bearing the burden of
financial cost, there would always be the possibility of moral hazards.[3]

Information on correct use of drugs

Most countries now require that manufacturers provide a package insert
for drugs which state the indications for prescription, warnings of adverse
effects, correct dosage and the price of the drug. Some countries produce
an independent annual publication which recommends specific drugs for
specific conditions (e.g. the *British National Formulary*). Finally, there are

Table 3.1 Daily dose of Amoxycillin by mouth recommended by Beecham in the UK and Germany

Age	Amoxil (Bencard, Subsidiary of Beecham, UK)	Clamoxyl (Beecham-Wüfing, Germany)
6–14 years	0.38–0.75 g	1.5 g
> 14 years	0.75–1.5 g	1.5–3 g

a number of national and international journals which give regular, independent evaluations of drugs or compare options for the treatment of common conditions. All of this information is based on the results of international clinical trials which compare the efficacy and safety of drugs. However, if this scientific evidence was the dominant influence on the drug market then there should be uniformity in prescribing habits. Some variation might be expected in the perceived drug of choice for a particular condition, but there should be uniformity of dosage for a specific drug. In fact manufacturers issue strikingly varying recommendations for the same drug in different countries as the following example shows.

Penicillins – an example of international variation in the drug market

Amoxycillin, a penicillin, is one of the most widely used antibacterial drugs in the world. The original patent was held by Beecham but has now expired so that other manufacturers are free to produce this drug. In the UK, amoxycillin is marketed by two manufacturers – Lagap and Bencard – which is a subsidiary of Beecham. There is also a third, non-proprietary formulation available. In Germany, amoxycillin is marketed by 16 different manufacturers[4] which implies that the German market is more lucrative than that of the UK. It is certainly bigger in terms of patient numbers but there are two other major differences – prices and dosage.

The price of 20 capsules of 500 mg amoxycillin from Beecham Wüfing (Germany) is 62–55 DM (roughly equivalent to £18.67 at current exchange rate), whereas Bencard, a subsidiary of Beecham, market the same product for £6.78. Presumably the price in the UK is pegged by the existence of a non-proprietary formulation of amoxycillin which, at £5.40 for 20 × 500 mg, is cheaper than the current UK Beecham price.[4]

Variations between countries in price for the same product might be expected particularly if a form of government control operates in one, but variations in dose are harder to explain yet they are almost as striking (See Table 3.1). The tablet/capsule strengths of amoxycillin marketed by Beecham in the UK are 0.25 and 0.5 g whereas in Germany they are 0.5, 0.75 and 1.0 g.[4]

This variation is by no means unique to amoxycillin or Beecham. For example, bacampicillin, another oral penicillin, is marketed by Upjohn at a dose of 0.8–1.2 g in the UK and 1.6–2.4 g in Germany.[4] In contrast, Japanese recommendations for daily dosage are much lower than in the UK because of different perceptions about toxic effects of penicillins. For example, clinical trials with Timentin (BRL 28500), a new penicillin, were conducted at a daily dose of 3.2–6.4 g in Japan (Fujimari and Mashimo, 1987), but 6.4–19.2 g in the USA and Europe (Robinson, 1987). Clearly, doctors' preconceptions about effective doses are completely different in these countries.

Efforts by Scottish Health Service managers[5] to improve efficiency

Since 1984, the need for efficiency improvement in the deployment of resources in the NHS in Scotland has been recognized. Ministers set up an 'Efficiency Programme Group' to determine priority areas in the NHS for review which were likely to yield resource savings. The Group presented their report in June 1985, listing a number of priority topics for review between 1985 and 1987. In order to take the review list forward, the group recommended the establishment of a Scottish Health Management Efficiency Group (SCOTMEG). Among the proposals was appropriate action on the distribution process from pharmacies to hospitals and community service.

SCOTMEG was established in September 1985 and a project was embarked upon in October 1985 to review the current process of supply and distribution of stocks from central pharmacies to hospitals and to the community service. The Action Plan was published in September 1987 and has subsequently been implemented throughout Scottish Health Boards. The general principles encompassed in the Action Plan were that:

(a) Formal mechanisms be established to facilitate variety reduction and assess and recommend products for inclusion in a formulary.
(b) Information systems be developed to provide finance and usage information to the prescribers.
(c) Full use be made of the professional skill of the pharmacists by creation of a ward pharmacy within Boards.
(d) Centralization of certain pharmacy services to be examined.
(e) Purchasing be strengthened by adoption of the most advantageous systems for each group of products and that prime wholesaler and sole vendor concepts be pursued.
(f) An integrated approach to all issues involved in pharmacy supply and distribution be adopted.

A further inquiry into purchasing has been established by SCOTMEG to develop a strategy on behalf of the Scottish Health Service for procurement, storage and distribution of medical products in order to achieve further improvement in procurement.

The general principles of the SCOTMEG Action Plan, as outlined above, may give the impression that the group has been mainly concerned with improvement of efficiency at Level 3 (purchasing, storage, and distribution). This impression is certainly wrong at Level 2 (prescription of medicine). The Scottish Health Service has also been well aware of the need for a formal mechanism to facilitate variety reduction and quality control and performance monitoring of the drugs. The specific suggestion to this end has been to set up a multi-disciplinary committee to recommend policies for the rational use of drugs. These should include:[6]

The development of policies for the use of medicinal products.
The production of a local formulary, and the updating and review of such a formulary.
The pursuit of safety and economy in the use of medicinal products and the control of their introduction.
The monitoring of the impact on patient care and the local formulary.

It was also suggested that the work on these committees could be aided by the establishment of specialist groups to undertake detailed studies on combining the economic efficiency and clinical choice together. Indeed, at least one such subcommittee is already functioning in the Tayside area. The Antibiotic Policy Group is a multi-disciplinary team of paediatricians, physicians, surgeons, a pharmacist and an economist who regularly meet to monitor the local pattern of antibiotic resistance and toxicology and prices of alternative drugs. The team is also actively involved in developing an appropriate methodology to influence prescribing.

Establishment of drug and therapeutics committees is a major step forward towards rationalization of the dose of individual drugs, not least because they remove psychological and actual barriers which the doctors would encounter if they act on their own. It takes a courageous doctor to alter the *status quo*, particularly if it involves a reduction in treatment from 'standard practice'. However, the successful introduction of reduced daily doses of a penicillin (mezlocillin) with considerable financial savings and no apparent harm to the patients has been described (Briceland *et al.*, 1988). This type of experimental approach is feasible in an academic centre where the academic has built a system for measurement of outcome financed by research funding. In contrast, a non-academic has no incentive to conduct this type of experiment and would inevitably argue that they have insufficient resources. Even a plea that a doctor should examine his/her current practice in relation to published literature is likely to be met with the excuse of 'insufficient time'. Doctors are too busy looking after patients to find out how to look after them properly.

As a first step towards rationalizing prescribing, we require more information about current prescribing habits. The late Professor Crooks conducted a survey on the use of barbiturates as sedatives by general practitioners in Tayside. Predictably, major differences were found and the survey was followed by a simple statement that barbiturates should be replaced by safer drugs and that the targeted prescriber was using proportionately more barbiturates than his/her peers. The result was very successful (Crooks, 1983) and other studies have convincingly demonstrated the efficacy of peer pressure in altering clinical practice (Fowkes *et al.*, 1986). The important point here is that it is not necessary to define optimum treatment; as a first step it is reasonable to define the average and try to compress the outliers of the market towards that.

It is extremely difficult to obtain accurate information on the drug market. The pharmacy in Tayside Health Board is being computerized and we are at least able to compare prescribing practices on different wards in order to highlight potential areas of wastage. However, we have no means of comparing our practice with another UK hospital, let alone with another country. The pharmaceutical industry employs an organization called Intercontinental Medical Statistics to provide information on the market differences but this information is not available to individual prescribers or even to drug formulary committees.

Improving collection and availability of information on national and international clinical practice should be a priority. Even crude information on drug prescribing habits would be valuable but, in the long term, a system is required which defines the condition treated and the outcome of treatment in sufficient detail to allow comparison of clinical practice.

To return to the intravenous penicillins, experts have stated in print that differences between certain penicillins are so marginal that doctors should use the cheapest available (Wise, 1982). Competitive tendering would take this a stage further, i.e. manufacturers might be asked to bid for an exclusive contract for a hospital for one year. However, in a recent experiment of this type in Tayside, manufacturers tendered linked bids. That is, where they could not compete on price for the market under discussion, they offered a package where an exclusive contract for one drug was linked to attractive discounts on other quite different drugs in use by the hospital. Linking of products in this way adds another level of complexity to the market.

As was stated earlier, at Level 3 of Fig. 3.2 is Pharmacy, and this is the section of the NHS with the unhappy task of bridging the gap between the commercial requirement of health managers and the clinical freedom of the doctors. It is interesting that while coming under stringent external financial pressure over the last decade or so, this is the section which has been most dynamic in both spotting the weakest links and coming up with some suggestions for improvement.

Over the last 20 years the most significant development in hospital pharmaceutical services has been the move of pharmacists out of the pharmacy on to the wards (Nuffield Foundation, 1986). The interface between Level 2 and Level 3 has been bridged by the emergence of specialized pharmacists working in the clinical setting, whose *raison d'être* is to assist the prescriber in the safe, effective and economic use of medicine by optimizing pharmaceutical factors which will help promote the desired response in the patient.

The success of programmes designed to improve efficiency at both Levels 2 and 3 will depend ultimately on the availability of two prerequisites. Firstly, a certain degree of financial autonomy at the area level should give them budgetary independence to plan and regulate their procurement on an annual basis. This would allow them, for example, to negotiate an early settlement discount with drug companies if the opportunity arises, or reduce the amount of stocks held by utilizing the Just In Time (JIT) concept, thus reducing the cost considerably. At the moment there is little incentive to reduce inventory holdings, although some of the pharmacists have already made considerable progress in that direction. For example, inventory holdings measured in terms of Days on Hand Forward (DOHF) in Tayside Health Board Area in July 1988 was 32.6 days, a figure well comparable to that of manufacturing industry. The implementation of the JIT concept will improve on these figures, but there should be some incentive to do this and present financial and budgetary arrangements are not conducive to these improvements.

The second prerequisite for implementation of efficiency programmes is the availability of good management information. Six of the Scottish Health Boards have installed the Pharmacy Supplies and Information System (PSIS) while other Boards have developed other pharmacy computer stock control and information systems. One Board is currently developing a pharmacy module as part of the Scottish Supplies Systems (SCOTSIS).

Conclusion

The experience of the Scottish Health Services shows that, faced with exogenous constraints beyond their control, health managers have increasingly become inward looking. In doing so, no significant improvements in performance and internal economies have accompanied major organizational and behavioural changes at local level. It is true that there is still an irreconcilable chasm between the concepts of 'efficiency' used by these managers and those of the central government but these differences by their very nature are political and they would never be settled on economic grounds. Looking for value for money and use of technology has been especially noticeable at pharmacy level. Information gathered at pharmacy level and involvement of the hitherto under-utilized resources of clinical pharmacists eventually will result in more efficient prescription practices. Future pharmacy information systems should be developed as part of clinical information systems to enable drug utilization data to be linked with patient data. This would provide quantitative data required for cost–effect evaluation of medicines in diagnostic related groups, and also facilitate the development of pharmacoepidemiology (Lawson, 1984).

A word of warning may be in order. As ward resource budgeting is introduced there is a danger that clinicians are swamped with computer-generated information which may remain unread. It is important that drug expenditure and utilization information should be concise and address the needs of the clinicians to allow them to make resource arrangement decisions.

Notes

1 See Maynard and Ludbrook (1980), p. 29. Our emphasis added.
2 Maynard (1980), p. 28. On the same recurrent theme, see also Culyer (1972), Maynard (1979), Maynard and Ludbrook (1980), Drummond (1981). For a slightly less sympathetic view see Lees (1966) and Green (1986).
3 See McLachlan and Maynard (1982), p. 559.
4 These included: Fischer, Stadapharm, Riker, Ratiopharm, Azuchemie, Beiendorf-Tüblinen, Wolff, Engelhard, Grünenthal, Beecham-Wüfing, TAD, Durachemie, Krewel, Pantorgan, Siegfried, Inpharzam. All data on German amoxycillin price and dose are from *Rote Liste 1988*, Bundesverband der pharmazeutischen Industrie CV, Postfach, Karlstrasse 21, 6000 Frankfurt A.M. (Editio Cantor, Aulendort/Wurtt, 1988). All data on UK amoxycillin price and dose from *British National Formulary*, No. 15, British Medical Association and the Pharmaceutical Society of Great Britain, 1988.
5 We use the term managers in the broadest sense to include doctors and pharmacists as well as the administrators.
6 Scottish Health Management Efficiency Group (SCOTMEG) (1987), p. 7.

References

Briceland, L.E., Nightingale, C.H., Quintiliani, R. and Cooper, B.W. (1988) Multidisciplinary cost-containment program promoting less frequent administration of injectable mezlocillin. *American Journal of Hospital Pharmacy*, **45**, 1082–5.
Crooks, J. (1983) Drug epidemiology and clinical pharmacology: their contribution to patient care. *British Journal of Clinical Pharmacology*, **16**, 351–7.
Culyer, A.J. (1972) On the relative efficiency of the National Health Service. *Kyklos*, **XXV**, 266–87.
Drummond, M.F. (1981) Welfare economics and cost benefit analysis in health care. *Scottish Journal of Political Economy*, **28**(2), June, 125–45.
Fowkes, F.G.R., Evans, K.T., Hartley, G., Nolan, D.J., Roberts, C.J., Davies, E.R., Green, G., Hugh, A.E., Power, M. and Roylance, J. (1986) Multicentre trial of four strategies to reduce use of a radiological test. *Lancet*, **1**, 367–70.
Fujimari, I. and Mashimo, K. (1987) Summary of clinical trials on BRL 28500 in Japan (clavulanic-ticarcillin). In: *International Symposium, Singapore, 13 February 1986*, Robinson, O.P.W. and Ferris, M.J. (eds), pp. 159–71. London: Medicom.

Green, D.G. (1986) *Challenge to the NHS*. Hobart Paperback no. 23. London: Institute of Economic Affairs.

Langle, L. *et al*. (1985) Le count d'un nouveau médicament. *Journal d'Economique Médical*, **2**.

Lawson, D.M. (1984) Pharmacoepidemiology: a new discipline. *British Medical Journal*, **289** (October).

Lees, D.S. (1966) *Economic Consequences of the Professions*. Research Monograph, no. 2, London: Institute of Economic Affairs.

McLachlan, G. and Maynard, A. (1982) The emerging lessons. In: The *Public/ Private Mix in Health Care*. McLachlan, G. and Maynard, A. (eds), pp. 513–58. London: Nuffield Provincial Hospitals Trust.

McLachlan, G. and Maynard, A. (eds) (1982) *The Public/Private Mix for Health*. London: Nuffield Provincial Hospitals Trust.

Maynard, A. (1979) Pricing, Insurance and the National Health Service. *Journal of Social Policy*, **8**(2) April, 157–76.

Maynard, A. and Ludbrook, A. (1980) What's wrong with the National Health Service? *Lloyds Bank Review*, no. 138, October, 27–41.

Nuffield Foundation (1986) Pharmacoepidemiology: emerging roles for pharmacists. *American Journal of Hospital Pharmacy*, **42**, April.

Robinson, O.P.W. (1987) Summary of clinical trials on BRL 28500 in Europe, UK and USA. In: *International Symposium, Singapore, 13 February 1986*, Robinson, O.P.W. and Ferris, M.J. (eds), pp. 172–9. London: Medicom.

Scottish Health Management Efficiency Group (SCOTMEG) (1987) *Review of Pharmacy Supply and Distribution Procedures*. Edinburgh: SCOTMEG.

Wise, R. (1982) Penicillins and cephalosporins: antimicrobial and pharmacological properties. *Lancet*, **2**, 140–43.

4 | Time and the Consultant: Issues of Contract and Control

Ken Starkey

Historically, the employment contract has functioned as an important mechanism in the development of managerial control. The dominant trend has been towards closed contracts with increasingly tightly specified temporal parameters. Some occupational groups have resisted this trend. Professionals have been particularly opposed to the application of the equation 'time is money' to the services they provide and the time they spend with their clients. Currently however, professional groups employed by the state are under attack on the grounds of accountability. Accountability is conceptualized by employers in terms of an adequate return on the time professionals are obliged, by contract, to commit to their work. It is associated with the framing of performance measures that depend on the commodification of time and the monitoring of time commitments made explicit by increasingly closed contracts.

This chapter examines the issues of time, contract and commodification as they apply to hospital consultants and general practitioners. It adds to Fox's view of contract as a managerial device aimed at 'the redefining of roles in terms of minimum discretion' (Fox, 1974, p. 62) the use of formal contract by occupational groups as an industrial relations weapon. Reference to contract by occupational groups can be used as a strategy for controlling the wage–effort bargain (Baldamus, 1961), especially in situations where the openness of contract is felt to leave the group open to abuse. In this situation there is a tendency to militate for greater closure of contract. The author questions whether this particular strategy is likely to be in an occupational group's best interest, suggesting with Fox that the gains of formally closed contracts are likely to be asymmetrical and in employer's/management's favour in the long run.

Hospital consultants

A generalized dissatisfaction among hospital consultants with the way their time was organized came to a head in the contract dispute of the 1970s between consultants and their ultimate paymaster, the government, represented by the then Department of Health and Social Security (DHSS). The medical profession came under pressure to accept a form of closed contract which it managed to resist (Castle, 1980). It was an interesting feature of this dispute, with a then Labour Government, that the profession put forward an alternative form of closed contract, although the nature of this closure differed from that sought by the DHSS. The profession argued that it was faced with a unique set of problems caused by the nature of its contract. Instead its spokesperson argued for a greater definition of the contracted time commitment on the part of their members. This demand arose partly through the feeling among many part-timers that they were being exploited by being required to provide a service as great as full-timers at a substantially lower salary. Some full-timers also found the demands made upon them were increasing steadily (BMA evidence to the Review Body on Doctors' and Dentists' Remuneration, *British Medical Journal*, 1979, p. 1653). The demand led to a confrontation between consultants and the Government. Central to the dispute were differing definitions of the relevant time commitments consultants should bring to their work; central to these definitions was the concept of clinical responsibility. Arguments revolved around whether this should be of an open or closed form, that is, all-embracing or limited to set, contracted times. Other grades of doctor were also dissatisfied with time aspects of their work. While the consultant dispute continued, junior hospital doctors went as far as taking strike action over hours of work which were, they argued, 'reminiscent of the nineteenth century' (Gordon and Iliffe, 1977, p. 6).

Consultants, too, argued that the existing open-ended contract with no specified time parameters, only an open commitment to total responsibility for the patients under their care, was no longer appropriate to medical work. Arguments over this issue raged, not only between the consultants as a body and their paymaster (the DHSS), but between consultants themselves. A minority felt that demands for restrictions on time were reminiscent of trade union behaviour and were not appropriate to a profession whose necessary level of commitment could not be fitted into the standard hours of an industrial-type contract. The profession's official representatives, however, were not averse to flexing their 'industrial muscle' as 'the only way if doctors are to keep afloat in today's inflationary society' (Gordon and Iliffe, 1977, p. 41). The goal was, if not a closed contract, then one that was more work-sensitive in its remuneration than the open variety. A contract that was closed enough to permit a large increase in pay would enable many members of the profession to regain the differentials that it had lost in previous pay-bargaining rounds. The

DHSS wanted a contract that was closed on its terms, specifying a Monday to Friday 9 a.m. to 5 p.m. week of 10 4-hour sessions rather than the Notional Half Days (NHDs) then specified in consultants' contracts (*British Medical Journal*, 4 January 1975, p. 45). The DHSS felt that some consultants, particularly the part-timers, were not fulfilling their obligations to the NHS and the new contract was designed to tighten management's ability to assert their control.

Monitoring the situation and trying to translate negotiation into pay recommendations was the Review Body on Doctors' and Dentists' Remuneration (the DDRB) which argued that professionalism and salaries related directly to length of working hours were incompatible: 'It is inappropriate to relate professional salaries to length of working hours' (Review Body on Doctors' and Dentists' Remuneration, 1977, para. 2.3). The maintenance of a binding ideology of professionalism was used in the Government's resistance to the junior doctors' collective action to achieve a new contractual status relative to time on the job. Gordon and Iliffe (1977) argue that the Government recognized the consequences of a dilution of the concept of professionalism would be that junior medical staff would no longer provide unpaid labour based solely on commitment to a professional career.

The consultants themselves clung to the notion of professionalism in their resistance to the Government version of a closed contract, arguing that the nature of professional work was incompatible with fixed hours, while at the same time holding the notion of professionalism in abeyance when it came to a close definition of the nature of their responsibilities in temporal terms. The DDRB argued that a set salary was the appropriate form of remuneration for professional work and that extra item-of-service payments and overtime-type payments were totally inappropriate. But the profession adopted a dual strategy, walking a fine line between claims for autonomy and the specification of 'out of hours' payments of the kind found in industry. Starting from the assertion that their earnings had seen a marked decline relative to other occupational groups they proceeded to link with this the argument that a large part of their work for the NHS was, in fact, voluntary and unpaid because it was conducted at times over and above their contracted hours. This they saw as an abuse of their good faith and used it as the basis of their pressing for a more closely defined contractual workload. As a form of action to support their case they proposed a 'work to contract'.

The new contract sought by the profession constituted a mix of sessional, emergency recall and on-call payments. It was to function in terms not of a timetable, 'with its spectre of clocking on and off' (Review Body on Doctors' and Dentists' Remuneration, 1978, para. 33) but according to a 'work schedule' over which the profession was to be the final arbiter. It differed from the old, open-ended contract in the extent to which aspects of the work previously covered by salary were to be separately contracted and paid for. It met the profession's three major objectives. Firstly, it limited the open-ended commitment of the old contract in defining what time commitment was covered and thus specifying when extra payments for extra duties were applicable, though the profession was explicit in stating that it did not regard 'the definition of individual contracts as synonymous with their closure' (*British Medical Journal*, 22 February 1975, p. 471). The consultant was still free to define when and what extra time was needed. Secondly, the contract guaranteed adequate remuneration for the NHS work by providing payment for work performed beyond contractual commitments. And, thirdly, it allowed consultants to do as they wished outside of their contracted hours. This time was now formally defined as 'free time'. The profession did not see this more precise definition of contractual responsibility as the abnegation or, indeed, any limitation of clinical responsibility or concern.

The Royal Commission on the NHS, though, expressed grave concern that the proposed contract constituted a step towards regarding work as an optional activity, as 'a favour to the patient rather than being part of the normal business of providing care'. It could thus be seen as subversive of the traditional consultant role of providing total care regardless of time (Royal Commission, 1979, para. 14:72). For the profession's negotiators it constituted, not a subversion, but, rather, an 'identification' of a standard working week against which extra time commitments could be measured and remunerated. It was not, they argued, a limitation of professional concern. The quality, and indeed, the quantity of care was not to be diluted. It was merely to be adequately remunerated.

Nevertheless, many influential members of the profession suggested that the proposed contract might constitute, in the long run, a Pyrrhic victory, facilitating a subsequent imposition of the dreaded closed contract. The profession would have to claim and justify overtime payments which would thus be open to administrative scrutiny. This could be construed as the first step towards the quantification of work and the specification of time norms for standard forms of activity which would eventually lead to the erosion of the professional freedom to allocate time to clinical, teaching, research and managerial activities as the individual consultant saw fit without interference from the employing authority. The door might thus be opened to the DHSS setting norms for the number of patients to be seen and treated per session and the regulation of treatment and discharge schedules (*British Medical Journal*, 1 January 1977, p. 53). The dispute in fact ended when a contract was offered and rejected by the profession at the eleventh hour on the grounds of its pricing schedule for consultants' services. The real reason for its rejection might have been that the profession did not want to leave itself more vulnerable to attempts to regulate its time in the future.

In the 1980s the question of contractual obligation arose again for two main reasons, firstly, with the Short Report and the avowed intention to reduce the number of doctors in junior medical grades. Consultants expressed concern that they would inevitably be faced with extra work as numbers in their teams were reduced. Secondly, there were problems in some authorities where management insisted that some elements of consultants' work, in particular on-call commitments, could not be considered as time worked and thus used to reduce commitments to work other clinical sessions. Some NHS authorities demanded that consultants complete work schedule diaries to demonstrate the nature of working patterns. The profession responded by stipulating what it considered a 'standard week'. Professional associations advised their members accordingly. The Hospital Consultants and Specialists Association was particularly militant here. The Faculty of Anaesthetists and the Royal College of Obstetricians and Gynaecologists went as far as setting out in writing norms for average working patterns in terms of such measures as operating sessions and patients per clinic.

The most significant proposal for hospital services in the 1989 White Paper *Working for Patients* is that of self-governing hospitals which would have delegated to them powers to provide services, to negotiate the price of services and to generate income. The major contractual implication of this proposal is that local hospital management would be free to determine pay and conditions of service for medical staff without reference to national agreements. This was opposed by the medical profession on the grounds that it is inconsistent with the principles of uniform standards within the NHS. Higher salaries in self-governing hospitals could lead to an uneven spread of high quality staff (BMA, 1989). The White Paper also argued for a more detailed job description for consultants to be reviewed annually with management. Job descriptions would include details of main duties, a weekly work programme, reference to participation in a medical audit, out-of-hours duties and management responsibilities. The profession argued that these proposals would offset the flexibility of the current contract. There was also the old objection that new managerial arrangements would cut into clinical time (BMA, 1989, para. 5.20):

> There is also the risk that unwieldy excessively bureaucratic procedures may result in a reduction in time available for clinical work. New job descriptions would need to take account of increased demand on consultants' time for management activities and audit, as well as traditional clinical commitments. If managers were to be closely involved in reviews of job descriptions, safeguards would need to be built in against narrow interpretations of contractual commitments, including rigid timetabling, inadequate recognitions of on-call duties, and reluctance to take account of non-district functions. Failure to provide such safeguards could result in a further adverse effect on the morale of consultants.

General medical practitioners (GPs)

The substantive implications of the White Paper for GPs are dealt with in detail in Chapter 5 but it is interesting to compare their contractual situation with that of hospital consultants. GPs remain independent contractors: instead of being paid a fixed salary for which they work an agreed number of hours, use premises, equipment, etc. provided by the employer, the contract is to provide general medical services to those patients who register with them. How, where and when it is done is to a large extent up to the doctor (Drury and Hill, 1979, p. 46). The GP, then, is not an employee of the Department of Health. An independent status has been jealously guarded by the profession precisely because it is considered to give GPs the freedom to organize the work which a salaried hospital doctor lacks (Royal Commission, 1979, para. 14.74). GPs thus enjoy considerable freedom to decide how to do their work and how much of their time to devote to patients – although their contract makes them responsible for 24-hour care, 365 days a year. This service does not have to be provided personally (Review Body on Doctors' and Dentists' Remuneration, 1982, p. 77).

General practice is seen as a business run 'if not for profit then at least to make ends meet' (Jeffreys and Sachs, 1984, p. 79). Income is based on a mix of capitation fees, a basic flat rate and seniority payments plus some item-of-service payments, for example, for night visits, immunization, cervical smears, and allowances for vocational and postgraduate training. GPs are also reimbursed for most of the salaries of ancillary staff such as receptionists. There is additional payment for group practice arrangements. Under special circumstances, where list size is small, payment may be more akin to a basic salary system as capitation fees would not provide adequate income. The contract is for services alone. It does not specify set periods of contracted time in the way of consultants. Nobody sets the GP's tasks or his or her timetable. GPs are free to organize these individually or among themselves in medical settings of their own creation.

Many changes occurred in general practice in 1965 with the so-called GPs' Charter. They reflected the fact that professionals had to set about managing their time better, because their new contracts specified responsibility for 24-hour care. The Charter paved the way for group practices and, thus, alleviated the responsibility of providing care single-handedly by the single GP. It also made available increased ancillary staff support. The changes signalled changes in professional attitudes among GPs. Later developments such as the widespread use of deputizing services testify to these. They are best exemplified in the work of the New Charter Working Group which published its demands for a radically restructured GP contract in 1979. Here an influential British Medical Association body set out how it would like to see the profession organized and its time commitments redefined. Its work has been construed as an exercise in reinterpretation of the traditional ethos of primary care. By limiting GPs' responsibility to their patients along a number of dimensions it predicates a reconceptualization of the concept of service.

The New Charter Group suggested a narrower definition of the GP's obligations with extra payment for services considered to be outside the normal bounds of duty (Wilding, 1982, p. 110). The Working Group argues that it is attempting to clarify ambiguity surrounding what constitutes a GP's duties and responsibilities as defined in the 1965 Charter. Part of its case is that a lack of agreed job specification has prevented the profession from using productivity deals concerning the provision of specified services as a means of pay bargaining. The contract in existence up until 1990 was an open-ended one with a GP getting limited pay for unlimited services. It called for greater use of fee-for-service payments as a means of making the contract more work-sensitive, arguing for a clear distinction between the GP's professional and ethical responsibility to the patient in providing continuing care and the additional contractual requirements of the NHS. The Group called for remuneration to be more closely linked to workload, particularly out-of-hours responsibilities, and a big reduction in list size to allow doctors more time for individual patients.

It is notable that the Group did not recommend either a totally salaried service (though some of its members called for this) or a total fee-for-service system. It wanted a greater use of fee-for-service payments and, implicitly, an end to the concept of the 'personal doctor' in the sense of a relationship between individual patient and doctor which binds the latter to a 24-hour day, a 7-day week, and all-year-round commitment. The Group concluded that the majority of the profession still wanted independent contractor status but with pay that reflected workload, skills and responsibility and reasonable working hours, with time for study and leisure, freedom from the contractual requirement of unending obligations to provide services personally and extra pay for work done outside the normal working day (General Medical Services Committee, 1983). The New Charter Group blamed deficiencies in on-going training among GPs on lack of time because courses are only available in leisure time. It argues for paid provision of time for study and professional development. The Group justified its aims by arguing that it was only following along a path already prepared by junior and senior hospital doctors. It is perhaps significant that the contract that was finally imposed on the GPs in April 1990 contained many features that might be seen to be in accord with the New Charter but with special payments weighted towards the communal duties (immunization, cervical smear testing, etc.) given priority by the then DHSS.

Implications

A key goal in the search for increased efficiency is the more intensive use of time reflected in the managerial imperative of extracting from time 'ever more available moments and from each moment ever more useful forces' (Foucault, 1979, pp. 151–2). Depending upon ideological stance, this search reflects exploitation (the Marxist perspective) or the march of rationalization (the Weberian view). Time is an essential element of the employment contract. Contracts, as they become more closed, tend towards increasingly explicit definition of temporal commitments reflecting 'the growing prevalence of the quantitative conception of temporality' (Zerubavel, 1981, p. 101). Dominant in Western industrial democracies is a commodified conception of time, epitomized in the saying 'time is money'. A consequence of such a conception is the quantification of time and efforts to organize social time in terms of economic production and profit. Time is always too short for management and too long for labour. Management tries to master time in order to prolong it while labour tries to master time in order to shorten it (Gurvitch, 1963, p. 44).

The work contract based on economic exchange is job-specific. It represents the power of management to impose its work designs. The worker 'supplies explicitly specified services' (Fox, 1974, p. 178). The effect of this explicitness is to curtail 'diffuse obligations'. The worker reacts to the low trust placed in him/her by refusing to give more than the contract stipulates. The formal contract, based on economic exchange, tends towards the maximum definition of what is expected of the employee whereas social exchange relations entail high trust relations based on unspecified obligations which are much more diffuse in their enactment, i.e. employees are prepared to give more as their side of the employment bargain. Social exchange depends on personal obligation, not impersonal rules, on discretion in an unsupervised work situation. Reciprocity is expected but it is not precisely defined as it is in economic exchange. The occupant of the high-discretion role participates in a community based on moral obligation not calculative expediency and pure market exchange (Fox, 1974).

Fox sees low-trust relations predominating in rank and file production work and contrasts this with professional work. The worker in the former 'has little sense of being an expert; of commitment to a calling; of autonomy on the job; or of obligation to produce high quality work; in other words, of being a professional' (Fox, 1974, p. 29). The specification of duties excludes choice which the professional retains. Professional obligations are diffuse. At present this diffuseness continues to be attacked by a reforming Conservative Government set upon redefining professional roles in terms of reduced discretion. But professionals themselves are anxious to limit what they consider the abuse of their professional commitment. In the consultants' dispute, one group of doctors moved towards contract because they felt their good will was being abused by their employers, yet finally they demonstrated an unwillingness to commit themselves to a less open contractual relationship, perhaps because of the control implications of such a move. GPs' aspirations have paralleled consultants' but as a group GPs have made major gains over the last quarter century in the amelioration of working conditions. Yet the New Charter Group can be seen to have formed a strategy that might be employed to bring about greater accountability by GPs.

Thus moves towards a more work-sensitive, 'closed' contract can generate unintended consequences. In further education, for example, a closed contract that was welcomed by lecturers in the 1970s as a major improvement in working conditions opened the door to the increased control of their working practices by local and national audit. By protesting too much, a profession can, like the queen in *Hamlet*, alert the outside world to the possibility that protest masks, if not guilt, at least a failure on its part to rationalize and improve the effective management of its time.

Conclusions

Fox suggests a link between stricter contractual relations and the erosion of trust between employer and employee. Both react to this erosion by moves towards more formally specified contract. Employers emphasize the obligations of contract, employees its limits. Moves towards a more detailed contract, by employers or employees, testify to a disequilibrium in the psychological contract. Employees subject to less discretion in their work and closer monitoring react by paying closer attention to the efforts they are willing to devote to it (Fox, 1974, p. 109):

> Accustomed to an assumption that they are giving maximum per-
> formance in the service of [organisational] ends . . . they find them-
> selves watched, measured, evaluated, and otherwise regulated by
> systematic, perhaps even quantitative, criteria. They reciprocate by
> reducing their commitment [to the organisation] and by weighing
> their contribution in a more calculative spirit.

The excuse of lack of time for not doing certain kinds of work can actually demonstrate a dwindling of commitment (Marks, 1977). A reduction in discretion leads to the alienation of self-estrangement and a diminution in the moral nature of the commitment to work (Fox, 1974, p. 83). Critics of professionals have discerned precisely this trend (Wilding, 1982). Pro-fessionals are not free of the 'calculative expediency' (Fox, 1974, p. 289) they criticize in others. Hence the movement towards a more detailed contract has been expedited by both sides.

One argument for the closure of contract is that the closed contract can function to make explicit the nature of exchange relationships between employer and employee. The move towards closure is motivated by a sense of inequities in exchange under open contractual arrangements. The problem of the use of contract as a solution to the perceived inequities of exchange arises mainly due to the use of contract for different ends by employers and employees. Under the present ideological opposition between employer and employed, a spontaneous move to common ground seems unlikely. Closed contracts have been linked to more explicit performance indicators, the rationale for which is that they will constitute a basis for judgement of the efficacy of service provision and the utilization of scarce resources. It remains to be seen how effective these performance indicators are in developing a rational approach to decision-making in the public services concerning the relationship between scarce resources and the public good. A major problem that the proponents of the use of such indicators have to resolve is that indicators might have unintended consequences for some client groups. In medicine, for example, they might favour treatment of a restricted group of patients with the most certain outcome and neglect of difficult cases (BMA, 1982). The immediate reaction to the fee-for-service system introduced for GPs in their 1990 contract on the part of some members of the profession has confirmed these fears. They have perhaps also served to confirm the existence of a 'calculative expediency' in the manner in which a minority of GPs have refused to continue to service clients rendered 'uneconomic' under the terms of their contract.

Professions are occupational groups who have been successful 'in the politics of today's work world' (Becker, 1971, p. 92). We seem to be witnessing a shift in power from professionals to the state which is, in the last analysis, the employer of the occupational groups examined here. The state has played an increasing role in the 'welfare compromise' (Hill, 1981, p. 247) that characterizes recent UK economic experience. The current economic situation is construed as the dysfunctional consequence of this compromise and a shift from concepts of social welfare to the needs of business is a major reaction to it. Critics of this development speak of the demise of the welfare state (Gough, 1979) as the sacrifice to counterbalance the 'fiscal crisis of the state' (O'Connor, 1973). Political contingency forces management to exert greater control over state employees (Batstone, 1984; Ferner, 1985). In professional work this would constitute a shift in the frontier of control (Storey, 1980, p. 125) away from professional auton-omy and an example of deprofessionalization. Some social theorists see deprofessionalization as the trend of the future and predict that pro-fessionals' control of their work will be challenged on its 'three basic dimensions of special knowledge, service and autonomy' (Haug, 1973, p. 199). It remains to be seen how the medical profession responds to the stronger managerial imperatives of financial stringency and control currently being voiced and whether its temporal autonomy can survive these pressures.

References

Baldamus, W. (1961) *Efficiency and Effort: An Analysis of Industrial Administration.* London: Tavistock.

Batstone, E. *et al.* (1984) *Consent and Efficiency: Management Strategy and Labour Relations in the State Enterprise.* Oxford: Blackwell.

Becker, H.S. (1971) *Sociological Work.* London: Allen & Unwin.

Castle, B. (1980) *The Castle Diaries, 1974–76.* London: Weidenfeld & Nicolson.

Drury, M. and Hill, R. (1979) *Introduction to General Practice*. London: Baillière Tindall.

Ferner, A. (1985) Political constraints and management strategies: the case of working practices in British Rail. *British Journal of Industrial Relations*, **23**(1), 47–70.

Foucault, M. (1979) *Discipline and Punish*. Harmondsworth: Penguin.

Fox, A. (1974) *Beyond Contract: Work, Power and Trust Relations*. London: Faber.

Gordon, H. and Iliffe, S. (1977) *Pickets in White: The Junior Doctors' Dispute of 1975*. London, MPU Publications.

Gough, I. (1979) *The Political Economy of the Welfare State*. London: Macmillan.

Gurvitch, G. (1963) *The Spectrum of Social Time*. Dordrecht: Reidel.

Haug, M.R. (1973) Deprofessionalization: an alternate hypothesis for the future. In: Halmos, P. (ed.) *Sociological Review Monograph*, no. 20.

Hill, S. (1981) *Competition and Control at Work*. London: Heinemann.

Jeffreys, M. and Sachs, H. (1984) *Rethinking General Practice*. London: Tavistock.

Marks, S.R. (1977) Multiple roles and role strain: some notes on human energy, time and commitment. *American Sociological Review*, **42**(6), 921–36.

O'Connor, J. (1973) *The Fiscal Crisis of the State*. London: St. Martin's Press.

Review Body on Doctors' and Dentists' Remuneration (1977) Seventh Report. London: HMSO.

Review Body on Doctors' and Dentists' Remuneration (1978) Eighth Report. London: HMSO.

Review Body on Doctors' and Dentists' Remuneration (1982) Twelfth Report. London: HMSO.

Storey, J. (1980) *The Challenge of Management Control*. London: Kegan Paul.

Wilding, P. (1982) *Professional Power and Social Welfare*. London: Routledge & Kegan Paul.

Zerubavel, E. (1981) *Hidden Rhythms: Schedules and Calendars in Social Life*. Chicago: Chicago University Press.

5 | The Future of Primary Care

Peter Bryden

Until the publication of the Government's White Paper *Working for Patients* and the controversy over the new contract for general practitioners, media discussion of the NHS had seemed inevitably to focus on the supposedly glamorous and high-tech world of hospital medicine with special emphasis either on revolutions in therapy or near-revolutions by one or other group of politicized employees. However, as the Government has recognized in the production of *Working for Patients* and in the subsequent Act, primary care services deal with over 90% of all episodes of ill health treated by the NHS. In addition, almost the entire workload of both the hospital in-patient and out-patient services originated in a referral from a general practitioner or primary health care team member – the only exceptions being those patients admitted to hospitals via the Accident and Emergency Departments, by the ambulance service or, very exceptionally, where patient self-referrals to certain specialized clinics were accepted.

Working for Patients recognized the gate-keeping or filtering role provided by general practitioners and sought to make the GP more responsible for control of this function by introducing indicative budgets for most practices together with fund-holding for those larger practices wishing to opt out of health authority control. As the document itself states – 'The GP will need to be aware in advance of the consequences for the budget of referral to hospital for diagnosis and treatment'.

The 1990 Act together with the new contract for GPs accelerated major role changes for both doctors and patients which have reflected national political and socio-economic changes since the inception of the NHS. The GP has metamorphosed from a professionally and managerially isolated healer of the sick, through to a member of the primary health care team during the decade or so when consensus-management was fashionable and on to the slick, efficient, competitive and highly audited provider of health care envisaged by the present Government.

Similarly, the patient has been transformed from a passive receiver of treatment, through the status of client with its implications of mutual discussion and respect, and on to the elevated position of consumer with the knowledge, ability and power to transfer his affiliation elsewhere should circumstances so dictate.

Throughout, however, the medical profession has clung to two basic tenets which have had profound influence on the management of primary care services – self-employed status for GPs by providing their services as independent contractors in contract with local Family Practitioner Committees (until 1974 known as Local Executive Councils), and personal registration of all NHS patients with one general practitioner who accepts responsibility for the provision of general medical services to every patient on his 'list' for 24 hours a day, 365 days per year.

The 1990 Act and the new contract entail much greater control, audit and outside influence by the health authority, by the Family Health Service Authority (replacing the Family Practitioner Committee), through peer review and through market forces, yet continuity is maintained by the retention of the self-employed status of the GP and by personal registration of patients.

Following the National Health Service Act (1946) prolonged and contentious discussions between the Government and the medical profession resulted in 1948 in the establishment of the NHS allowing GPs together with community-based dentists, pharmacists and opticians to retain their status as independent contractors. Contracts were initially held by Local Executive Councils which exercised a fairly limited management role. They ensured that contractors complied with their terms and conditions of service, they took responsibility for payments to these practitioners and they were also involved with inspection of premises, handling of complaints and selection of new entrants.

In addition, the Medical Practices Committee was established to attempt to achieve a more even distribution of GPs throughout the country. This body has the power to refuse permission for additional GPs in areas considered to be 'over-doctored' and to encourage, by inducement payments, more medical manpower into areas where average list size is high. However, by the end of the 1950s, this rather relaxed management style with clinically orientated, self-employed and mainly self-interested GPs running their own practices, usually from their own premises, with benign oversight but virtually no innovation or planning function from the Local Executive Councils, had led to stagnation, loss of initiative and a decline in the numbers of new entrants to general practice with consequent reversal of the fall in average list size. By the early 1960s the position was becoming critical and in the absence of positive leadership from the Government the medical profession itself undertook a review of the future direction of general practice. In 1965, the General Medical Services Committee of the British Medical Association presented to the Government a document entitled *A Charter for the Family Doctor Service*. This document has been the blueprint for the development of contemporary primary care. Several important concepts on which present-day general practice are based resulted from the *Charter*.

Certainly the most important development was the provision of reimbursement for expenditure on staff and premises. General practitioners were now able to claim reimbursement for 70% of the cost of ancillary staff and schemes for the reimbursement of rent and rates, together with the Cost Rent Scheme, enabled premises to be modernized, improved and enlarged. Amalgamation of smaller practices into larger units was encouraged by group practice payments available to practices of three or more principals. The GP was now working in larger groups or partnerships, from more sophisticated premises and with a larger number of ancillary staff. As the process evolved, GPs became the employers of a small but nevertheless often significant number of staff. Consequently, the doctors became responsible for substantial paperwork involving national insurance and income tax, pension contributions, employers' liability, etc. Some doctors were willing to perform these tasks personally but many opted out. Most practices delegated this work to a senior member of the ancillary staff, later to develop into the practice manager, whilst others had opted out entirely by electing to work from health authority-owned health centres where all staff were employed by the health authority. GPs who moved into health centres found that they were members of a team of health care workers based in one building. Very often community nurses, health visitors, chiropodists, community dentists and other community-based health care workers also worked from the same building. Community nurses, health visitors, community midwifes and sometimes social workers were usually attached to one practice or group of practices. Thus a number of primary health care workers employed by the health authority worked as a team with a group of self-employed GPs from health authority-owned premises. The receptionists, cleaners and other ancillary staff were also employed by the health authority. The primary health care workers and ancillary staff were responsible to their superiors in the health authority and not to the self-employed medically qualified members of the team. Thus the concept of a consensus-managed primary health care team with no definitive leadership had been achieved.

However, health centres were not particularly popular with GPs and in many areas GPs could not be encouraged to work from them. The perceived threats to the self-employed status of the doctor usually outweighed the benefits provided by provision of a building and ancillary staff. Nevertheless, those doctors who continued to practise from their own premises also saw the benefits of a team of health care professionals working together in a community. As new surgery premises were planned, and eventually built, accommodation came increasingly to be provided for fellow members of the primary health care team. It is now commonplace for health authority-employed community nurses, midwives and health visitors to work from premises owned by GPs, often in association with practice nurses employed by the practice.

Practice managers have also evolved from the senior receptionist who undertook 'a little paperwork', into a recognized profession with considerable responsibilities. Training courses and diplomas have been developed and many practice managers have become experienced in personnel management, book-keeping, contracts of employment for staff, forward planning, etc.

Another major contribution to primary care from the 1965 *Charter* was the emphasis on continuing post-graduate education for family doctors. The College of General Practitioners had been formed in 1952 to encourage GPs to undertake post-graduate education and to foster the development of such courses. In the 1965 *Charter* this important role was recognized and the College gained its Royal Charter two years later. The Todd Report on medical education was published in 1968 and recommended vocational training for general practice. Mandatory vocational training was introduced in 1982 and since that date all new GPs must have spent three years following their pre-registration hospital appointments in a combination of recognized hospital posts and attachments to one or more training practices.

Although since the 1965 *Charter* doctors have had considerable opportunity to improve and develop their practices, the cost of greater government involvement in contributions towards ancillary staff and reimbursement of rent and rates has been a higher profile governmental managerial role especially since the Local Executive Councils were replaced by the Family Practitioner Committees in 1974. The payments of basic practice allowance, item of service fees and other allowances such as seniority, vocational training and group practice allowance have involved increased monitoring of the services and facilities provided by the self-employed contractors. Ancillary staff payments and especially payments under the Improvement Grant or Cost Rent Scheme have involved prior approval before staff wage rates are increased or money is spent on improving premises, or building new premises. Increasingly frequently in recent years, Family Practitioner Committees have made interpretations on various paragraphs of the Statement of Fees and Allowances (the general practitioners' rule book) which have caused appeals to be made to the Secretary of State to adjudicate on their legality. This more robust management style on the part of Family Practitioner Committees has been even more apparent since the Government made clear its intentions towards primary care and the NHS as a whole.

The new Contract for General Practitioners introduced in April 1990 involved a considerably increased management role for the new locally contracting body, the Family Health Service Authority (FHSA). For the first time audited performance-related payments (rather than individual item of service payments) are offered for cervical cytology and childhood immunizations. Under this scheme, bonus payments are made for reaching targets. No payment is made for below-target performance. Lower rate and higher rate payments are offered for achieving lower and higher targets. FHSAs have powers to require GPs to live 'within a reasonable distance' from their surgeries – 'reasonable' to be defined by the FHSA – and there is a requirement to produce practice leaflets and an annual report. FHSAs also monitor GPs' hospital referral rates. In addition, there are incentives on offer in the form of financial inducements to perform minor surgery, child development surveillance, health promotion clinics and teaching of undergraduate medical students. The importance of capitation fees has been increased so that these fees make up approximately 60% of GPs' income rather than the approximately 46% previously, i.e. it has become financially more beneficial to accept a larger number of patients onto individual lists. Disincentives, in the form of lower pay rates, apply to the use of deputizing services to undertake out-of-hours calls.

The management implications of these Contract changes both to the FHSA and GPs are profound. The Family Health Service Authority has now to develop or improve systems to audit take-up rates for cervical cytology and childhood immunizations. There will need to be an adequately thought-out mechanism to deal with disputes over figures and an appeals procedure. Forward planning will be necessary to produce guidelines for acceptable practice leaflets and annual reports. Health promotion clinics run by practices have to be assessed with regard to acceptability for payments. The experience of GPs wishing to carry out child development surveillance and minor surgery sessions has to be established. Much greater use of computers will be essential to monitor referral rates and target payments. The old Family Practitioner Committees were not in the forefront with regard to the development of information technology in the NHS: it has yet to be seen what role their successors will adopt in this regard.

GPs will need to come to terms with the greatly increased power of government and the FHSAs to direct the way in which they work. Although the profession has been pressing for contract changes with regard to payment for child development surveillance and minor operations for some years and although medical audit has long been encouraged by bodies such as the Royal College of General Practitioners, target payments and performance-related pay are completely new concepts for many GPs. Practices will need to examine their methods of working in order to accommodate new clinical sessions whilst maintaining adequate routine surgery and home-visiting time. Although many practices are already computerized the large number without such systems will need to consider investment in information technology in order to obtain information on populations targeted for immunization, child surveillance, Well-Woman, Well-Man, cervical cytology, etc. Disease registers will be needed to identify groups such as diabetics, hypertensives and asthmatics for health promotion clinics.

Performance-related pay will necessitate information on cervical cytology and child immunization rates being accurately provided. GPs, especially if coping with an increased list following the changes to the proportion of income generated by capitation fees, will need to delegate a greater proportion of the workload. Delegation will be to practice nurses and specialized ancillary staff such as counsellors, but also possibly to doctors working as assistants rather than as full principals. The new contract allows for increased payments to employ an assistant. The primary health care team will therefore of necessity be expanded to include more GP-employed personnel and the practice nurse, nurse practitioner and assistant GP will all become more evident.

As the primary health care team expands, so also will the role of the practice manager. Increased planning and coordination will be necessary together with monitoring of progress towards targets and call-up of patients to health promotion clinics. The practice manager will almost certainly become responsible for the production of the practice leaflet and annual report. Personnel management and public relations, together with staff training, on-going audit, forward planning, coordination and communication with Family Health Service Authorities (FHSAs) and District Health Authorities will all fall into the practice manager's sphere. GPs will increasingly find that their own management role is diminished as those of the Family Practitioner Committee and the practice manager increase. Conversely, GPs will be able to devote more time to clinical work which will become more rigidly planned out.

GPs at first reacted defensively to these changes in their contract. In 1989 the Special Conference of Representatives of Local Medical Committees narrowly rejected the recommendation of the General Medical Services Committee to accept an agreement with the Secretary of State over the New Contract Proposals. The Government responded by imposing a contract on GPs.

Further and more fundamental changes were envisaged in the White Paper *Working for Patients*. The proposals contained in this document and in the subsequent Act are still being worked out in practice. However, the areas in which the future shape of primary care are being determined include indicative budgets for prescribing, practice budgets for larger practices, contracts for hospital services, medical audit and changes in the structure of FHSAs to come.

Under the new arrangements, indicative drug budgets are set for general practitioners by the FHSA. Normally budget levels are set at a figure corresponding approximately to average levels for that area but taking into account any local factors which may be relevant. For practices where current prescribing levels are above average, the indicative budget is set at a level between their current figure and the FHSA average for comparable practices in the same Authority area. According to the White Paper, over time these procedures will bring downward pressure to bear on those practices which have above average prescribing costs which cannot be explained by local factors. The White Paper states that, 'Divergence from the budget profile will indicate the need for action. Initially action will take the form of peer review or a request to the FHSA for help and guidance'. The Family Health Service Authority will monitor individual practices' performance against their indicative budgets and take appropriate action to maintain expenditure within the budget. The Authority was authorized to investigate 'any significant divergence of actual planned expenditure, together with any apparent cases of excessive prescribing'. Explanations are to be sought from the practice concerned and where thought necessary remedial action is to be taken. It is expected that this will take the form of discussion, probably involving independent medical advice, but where 'discussion, education and peer review' have no effect it will be open to FHSAs as a last resort to initiate action to take appropriate sanctions, the final outcome of which may be withholding of remuneration from the doctors concerned.

The subsequent Act has brought into being a significant minority of autonomous GP fund-holders. Their budgets cover hospital services such as surgical in-patient and day-case treatment, out-patient services and diagnostic investigations together with the costs of drugs, staff and certain costs relating to premises. The practices within this scheme receive their funds direct from the Regional Health Authority and are expected to stay within the agreed budget. Participating practices are able to decide for themselves where to refer patients to ensure the most effective use of their funds. They are free, within limits, to purchase services from District Health Authority managed hospitals, self-governing hospitals or the private sector. Over-spending of budgets is to be dealt with in a similar way to the mechanisms for prescribing budgets, i.e. the FHSA will initiate a thorough audit including advice from other doctors and overspending at a level greater than 5% for two years in succession may result in a practice losing the right to hold its own fund. Non-fund-holding practices usually refer patients to hospitals with which their local District Health Authority has negotiated a contract. Only in special circumstances are referrals to other hospitals accepted. (Before the Act GPs were free to refer patients to practically any consultant throughout the country.)

The composition of the local FHSAs (formerly Family Practitioner Committees) has also changed. The effect of this has been to considerably reduce professional representation on the Boards of FHSAs. Medical advice is to be sought from independent advisers and the role of the Local Medical Committee (a body elected by general practitioners and providing advice to the Family Practitioner Committee) has been considerably diminished as a result. In order to effectively cope with the changes envisaged in both the new contract and the Act, management of FHSAs has been considerably strengthened. General managers have been appointed.

Salary levels among recent appointments reflect a desire to attract candidates with suitable managerial skills and experience, with a view, perhaps, to avoiding a repetition of the unfortunate consequences of certain District Health Authority general manager appointments.

Understandably as a result of these considerable changes GPs at present feel threatened and anxious about their future. The advantages of independent contractor status have been seriously eroded and it is not surprising that the merits of a salaried service have begun to be discussed, albeit with little enthusiasm so far. Even the concept of personal lists could be under threat in the future as further changes in structure could well lead to developments such as health authorities 'buying' primary care services from groups of doctors rather than patients being registered on individual lists.

The future is difficult to predict. The Government, the opposition parties and the medical profession have already noted the effects of threats to the NHS on the electorate. There will be further confrontation, negotiation and debate. It is possible that the medium-term future of the NHS will not be entirely settled until after the next general election. However, it is also very likely that primary care will continue to become more tightly managed in the future, both by government and by practice management. Consumerism, efficiency and cost-effectiveness have become a way of life and are likely to remain so whatever the political shade of the next government. Primary care cannot be either insulated or isolated from these developments.

References

GMSC (1965) *A Charter for the Family Doctor Service*. London: General Medical Services Committee of the British Medical Association.

Health Departments of Great Britain (August 1989) *General Practice in the National Health Service: the 1990 Contract*. London: HMSO.

Royal Commission on Medical Education 1968, Report Appendix 19. London: RCME.

Secretaries of State for Health, Wales, Northern Ireland and Scotland (January 1989) *Working for Patients*. London: HMSO.

6 | Nurse Practitioners and the Changing Face of General Practice

Sheila Greenfield

Since the mid-1980s several important influences have combined to profoundly affect the face of general practice and it is now facing perhaps the biggest shake up since the NHS began 40 years ago. Contemporary social trends such as the growth of the elderly population, the pressures of redundancy and unemployment, the shift of patients from hospital to the community, increased awareness among the population of their needs and of preventive medicine, the replacement of acute infections as causes of morbidity and mortality by chronic degenerative diseases, are placing increasing demands upon the community and primary care services.

One of the ways in which general practice has attempted to respond to these changes has been to increase the number of practice nurses employed by general practitioners in their surgeries to help relieve them of much of the routine clinical work and to assist in preventative care and management of chronic disease. There has also been a growing trend for many tasks hitherto undertaken by GPs to be delegated to practice nurses.

The role of the practice nurse

The title 'practice nurse' has come to be applied to nurses who are directly employed by GPs and work mainly within treatment rooms in the practice buildings, professionally defined (*The Practice Nurse*, May, 1988, p. 5) as:

> A registered general nurse who is employed by the General Practitioner to work within the treatment room and is a member of the team responsible for the clinical nursing care of the practice population together with the district nursing team of the health authority.

Table 6.1 The role of the practice nurse

Disease and illness prevention	*Screening as a function of primary care*
Health education	Screening patients new to the practice
Preconceptual care	Well woman clinic
Parentcraft	Young adults' health checks
in early pregnancy	Elderly patients' health checks
in the second trimester	Preretirement group
in the third trimester	Child development and surveillance
Postnatal group	clinics
Clinics for special groups of patients	*In the treatment room*
Antenatal	Designing
Postnatal	Planning
Family planning	Maintenance and management
Baby and toddler	Purchasing and maintaining equipment
Obesity	Stock control
Blood pressure	Procedures and techniques for use in
Diabetic	the treatment room
Stop smoking	
Immunization	
Vaccination	
Administration of the practice	*Research*
Communication	Practice studies
Staff training	Studies in conjunction with the Medical
Implementing legislation, such as the	Research Council and projects such
Health and Safety at Work Act	as the Oxford Prevention of Heart
	Attacks and Stroke Project
	Studies in conjunction with hospitals on
	topics such as nocturnal asthma and
	testicular carcinoma

The role of the practice nurse is wide ranging and according to Jeffree (1988) can include the activities listed in Table 6.1.

Although the journal *The Practice Nurse*, which appeared for the first time in May 1988, comments (p. 5) upon the rapid expansion in the number of practice nurses, an increase of 120 per cent since 1979 to about 5000 today, the practice nurse is by no means a newcomer to the surgery. As Bowling (1981b) states: 'Since 1911, at least one general medical practice in England has employed a nurse continually.' A further milestone was reached in the mid-1960s when GPs were allowed to reclaim 70 per cent of ancillary staff salaries and to delegate tasks to nurses. However, it is only since 1986 that practice nurses have really made their presence felt both in terms of their number and in the way they have succeeded in making their collective voice heard.

Since the mid-1960s a number of studies have looked at various aspects of the role of the practice nurse. Case studies of individual practices (Cartwright and Scott, 1961), the practice nurse's suitability to undertake first home visits to patients, their social and occupational characteristics (Reedy *et al.*, 1980a and b) and delegation of medical tasks to nurses have been explored (Bowling, 1981 and 1987). It is this last mentioned aspect of the practice nurse's work that has been the focus of much attention since 1990. As the primary health care team has expanded so has the number and variety of procedures undertaken by practice nurses. This was demonstrated by a study (Greenfield *et al.*, 1987) in the West Midlands which showed that whilst the majority of practice nurses performed traditional nursing tasks (measuring blood pressure, removing sutures, giving injections, applying dressings and syringing ears), 70 per cent carried out cervical smears, almost two-thirds were undertaking breast and vaginal examination, and a number of them diagnosed, investigated and treated common ailments. The study also revealed that the majority of nurses thought that, with appropriate training, they could carry out a wider range of tasks than they do at present (Tables 6.2 and 6.3). Comparison with the activities of nurses in Reedy's 1977 study (Reedy *et al.*, 1980b) indicates to what extent the role of the practice nurse is developing (Tables 6.4 and 6.5). This trend has raised the question as to whether a role similar to that of the nurse practitioner in the USA is desirable or appropriate for general practice in the UK.

The practitioner concept

A nurse practitioner, then, is a highly trained nurse who in addition to carrying out routine nursing duties can act as a first contact for patients and perform some of the general practitioner's duties such as diagnosing illness. The term 'nurse practitioner' was first used in the USA during the mid-1960s when nurses who worked in primary health care began to extend their role sometimes acting as substitute medical practitioners in rural and inner city areas where the provision of medical care was inadequate (Reedy, 1978). Studies in the USA which have assessed the safety and effectiveness of nurse practitioner care have found that it can compare satisfactorily with that provided by doctors (Spitzer *et al.*, 1974) and in certain areas such as lowering blood pressure, weight reduction and complying with treatment nursing care can even be more effective (Ramsay *et al.*, 1982; Watkins and Wagner, 1982).

The possible potential of this concept for primary care in the UK was highlighted in three recently published discussion documents aimed at improving the quality of primary care. The Government's Green Paper *Primary Health Care – An Agenda for Discussion* (Secretaries of State for Social Services, April 1986), closely followed by its White Paper *Promoting Better Health* (Secretaries of State for Social Services, 1987) and the (then)

Table 6.2 Tasks which practice nurses currently performed and those which nurses thought they should do or could do with appropriate training

Task	Percentage of nurses currently performing*	Percentage of nurses who think they should/could perform*
Measurement of blood pressure	96.3	86.7
Suture removal	95.3	87.9
Intramuscular injection	94.9	87.6
Subcutaneous injections	94.6	88.0
Application of suitable dressings	93.9	88.0
Ear syringing	93.3	87.1
Intradermal injections	81.6	86.4
Venepuncture for blood sampling	74.5	87.2
Cervical smears	70.5	87.0
Auroscopic examination of ears, nose and throat	67.8	88.0
Examination of breasts	62.0	88.0
Speculum examination of vagina and cervix	60.0	85.7
ECG recordings	57.0	89.2
Referral of patients to other members of primary health care team, social services and local voluntary agencies	55.3	81.6
Assistance at or initiation of resuscitation until medical help is obtained	55.0	91.6
Observation of skin for signs of disease	52.5	85.4
Measurement of respiratory function	50.3	85.0
Examination of bones and joints	39.9	65.8
Intrauterine device removal	18.0	55.3
Psychological examination for early signs of anxiety and depression	13.0	49.8
Bimanual examination of uterus and adnexae	10.7	42.1
Ophthalmoscopic examination of eyes	9.0	51.4
Stethoscopic examination of heart and chest	7.6	47.2
Palpation of abdomen	4.3	26.5
Palpation of liver, kidneys and spleen	2.6	19.0
Examination of penis and testicles	2.3	31.7
Referral of patients to consultants	2.3	12.4

* Total number of responses varied for each item (from 291 to 297)
Source: Journal of the Royal College of General Practitioners (1987) **37**, p. 342–3.

Table 6.3 Problems which practice nurses were currently involved in managing and those which nurses thought they could manage with appropriate training

Problem	Percentage of nurses currently managing*	Percentage of nurses who think they could manage*
Uncomplicated minor injuries (sprains, simple abrasions and cuts)	69.8	89.4
Hypertension	52.0	80.0
Simple allergies (hay fever or insect bites)	46.8	80.3
Family planning advice	36.1	80.0
Common infectious diseases	34.7	79.9
Urinary tract infections in women	30.4	68.3
Vaginal discharges	30.4	63.4
Conjunctivitis	29.7	73.0
Diabetes	28.8	70.7
Monilial infections of the mouth	25.7	77.0
Otitis externa	25.0	69.7
Seborrhoeic dermatitis of scalp and mild eczema	22.7	71.0
Upper respiratory tract infection including tonsillitis	20.8	60.9
Acute otitis media	19.3	50.5
Asthma	16.1	52.9
Rheumatic diseases	10.7	43.6
Thyroid disease	9.7	38.9
Mild heart failure	8.0	33.0

* Total number of responses varied for each item (from 291 to 297)
Source: Journal of the Royal College of General Practitioners (1987) **37**, pp. 342–3

DHSS *Community Nursing Services and Primary Health Care Teams* (DHSS, 1987), all emphasized the following objectives:

- to make primary health care services more responsive to the needs of the consumer
- to raise standards of care
- to promote health and prevent illness
- to give patients the widest range of choice in obtaining high-quality primary care services
- to improve value for money
- to enable clearer priorities to be set for Family Practitioner Services in relation to the rest of the NHS.

Table 6.4 'Intermediate' activities (for nurses or doctors) of attached and employed nurses (percentages)

	Attached nurses		Employed nurses	
	Activities Ever done	Activities Done in last month	Activities Ever done	Activities Done in last month
Surgical dressings of all kinds	100	93	85	80
Tested urine	97	94	94	93
Removed sutures	96	87	86	76
Measured temperature, pulse, and respiration	92	91	74	72
Given counsel or support	91	87	84	75
Adjusted slings or dressings	89	77	80	73
Given eye treatments	83*	69	49	38
Catheterized a patient	77*	64	17	7
Changed vaginal pessaries	65*	51	33	20
Taken swabs for bacteriological examination	64	45	63	59
Given preventive inoculations (except smallpox)	50*	29	96	90
Weighed patients	45*	41	84	75
Taken blood pressure	40*	29	78	69
Performed dip-slide culture on urine	25*	22	49	43
Removed plaster of Paris	8	4	5	3
Performed biochemical tests on faeces	5	2	2	0
Performed audiometry	4	2	0	0

* Differences between the proportion of nurses who had 'ever done' the activity are significant beyond the one per cent level
Source: *Journal of the Royal College of General Practitioners* (1980) **30**, pp. 484–5

A fundamental element in this process is seen to be the need for an extended role for the nurse in primary care and for increased numbers. In the Green Paper (DHSS, 1986, p. 18):

> We would like to see ... the introduction into primary care of the nurse practitioner. She would work alongside doctors, would be responsible to them for agreed medical protocols and be available for direct consultation by patients.

And in the White Paper (Secretaries of State for Social Services, 1987, p. 16):

> The introduction of *nurse practitioners* into primary care was well supported .... The Government welcomes the interest shown in the

Table 6.5 'Technical' activities (traditional medical) of attached and employed nurses (percentages)

	Attached nurses		Employed nurses	
	Activities Ever done	Activities Done in last month	Activities Ever done	Activities Done in last month
Syringed ears	53*	40	82	79
Performed venepuncture for laboratory specimens	24*	22	47	43
Carried out specific desensitizing procedures	24	20	35	35
Incised boils and abscesses	16*	10	58	46
Applied plaster of Paris or cervical collar	13	9	20	18
Taken and prepared cervical smears	11*	5	39	37
Vaccinated against smallpox	11*	6	35	35
Performed electrocardiographs	9*	4	26	25
Cauterized wounds etc.	9*	2	40	34
Carried out skin testing with allergens	8	4	13	9
Performed pregnancy tests	4*	2	20	19
Estimated haemoglobin	4	4	15	11
Inserted sutures after injecting local anaesthetic	4*	2	32	26
Set up and read ESR	4	2	16	11
Used peak flow meter	2*	0	18	18
Fitted IUCD	2	2	2	2

* Differences between the proportion of nurses who had 'ever done' the activity are significant beyond the one per cent level
Source: Journal of the Royal College of General Practitioners (1980) **30**, pp. 484–5

concept and intends to look further at such issues as legal status, functions and qualifications. (author's emphasis)

In view of the amount of attention that the concept of the nurse practitioner has received, it is surprising that there have been so few attempts to systematically test the role out in practice in this country. In some settings, patients have been allowed open access to practice nurses (Cartwright and Anderson, 1981) and the study of the social and occupational characteristics of 300 practice nurses carried out by Greenfield *et al.* (1987) revealed that a number of practice nurses felt that the extended way in which they were working resembled in many respects the role of a nurse practitioner. However, as the title of 'nurse practitioner' is not yet formally recognized by the Royal College of Nursing (RCN), there are no figures for the number of nurses working as 'nurse practitioners' in the

UK nor indeed any formal definition of the role. The doubt and confusion that surround this issue were underlined by the Royal College of Nursing's nurse adviser to the Society of Primary Health Care who commented that many practice nurses had written to the RCN in the belief that they were nurse practitioners. She emphasized however that (Jesop, 1986, p. 20):

> There is no way you can become a nurse practitioner without training. There is a lack of understanding of what being a nurse practitioner entails.

Two small practical studies do nevertheless exist which have used the US model as their basis. In the first of these (Reedy *et al.*, 1980c) a final-year US physician's assistant was attached to a health centre in Reading for eight weeks and managed 221 cases under supervision (Table 6.6). It appears that the doctors in the practice felt that the experiment had worked well and had been very acceptable to patients, but both doctors and nurses in the practice were doubtful whether this type of physician's assistant would be appropriate for general use in the UK.

A more recent study (Stilwell *et al.*, 1987) designed to examine the role a nurse practitioner based on the US model could play in a UK general practice took place in the West Midlands between 1982 and 1985. In this study the nurse, to whom patients had open access, was based in an inner-city general practice in Birmingham and the characteristics of the 858 patients who consulted her during a six-month period and the nature of their consultations were recorded. The study concluded that nurses could indeed play a much larger and more autonomous part in the care of patients than they do at present. Patients from all ages and ethnic groups in the practice consulted the nurse practitioner about problems from every diagnostic group (Royal College of General Practitioners and Office of Population Censuses and Surveys, 1981) although most were of a preventative, educational, social or administrative nature (see below). Patients tended to direct themselves to the nurse practitioner with problems appropriate for her skills and in more than one-third of cases she was able to manage the problem herself without the need for further referral. As a result of her experiences in this study, Barbara Stilwell (1985, p. 155), the nurse practitioner involved concluded that:

> A nurse who is adequately prepared can competently carry out health checks on men and women aged between 19 and 60 which include the following:

Examine	*Lifestyle*	*Discuss and Teach*
Blood pressure	Smoking	Testicular self-
Heart, chest and	Diet	examination
abdomen	Exercise	Breast self-
Peak expiratory	Alcohol	examination
flow rate	consumption	

Table 6.6 Primary diagnosis of patients seen by the physician's assistant

Diseases	International classification	Episodes		Second national morbidity survey %
		No.	%	
Respiratory system	460–519	27 }	29	22
Hay fever/allergic rhinitis	407	38 }		
Skin subcutaneous tissues	680–709	23	10	8
Musculoskeletal and connective tissues	712–739	17	8	6
Genitourinary system	580–629	16	7	5
Ear	380–387	13	6	4
Infective and parasitic	008–136	12	5	4
Digestive system	520–578	10	5	4
Circulatory system	390–458	8	4	5
Accidents, poisoning, and violence	N802–994	7	3	6
Pregnancy, childbirth and puerperium	{ Y60–62 } { 631–678 }	6	3	9
Mental disorders, central nervous system, and eye	294–378	5	2	12
Neoplasms	151–239	4	2	1
Endocrine, nutritional, and metabolism	240–279	< 1	1	2
Physical symptoms and signs	780–	10	5	10
Miscellaneous conditions	Y00–99 (except Y60–62)	24	11	2
Totals		221	100	100

Source: British Medical Journal (1980) **230**, p. 655

Examine	*Lifestyle*	*Discuss and Teach*
Cholesterol levels	Stress	
Urine testing, height, weight, cervical cytology	Particular concerns Family history of cardiovascular disease	

Consumer response

The behaviour of patients in the above study perhaps tends to reflect the increase in awareness about the role of nurses in the surgeries of general practitioners highlighted in a recent report by *Which* (1987) in which both consumers' and providers' views of primary health care services were sought. It revealed that from the patients' point of view the most important service which helps to make a 'good practice' is the availability of a practice nurse. This contrasts with the results of the Marplan Poll (1985) carried out in 1985 for the Community Nursing review team which showed that only 10 per cent of people interviewed knew anything about the role of the practice nurse. During the Birmingham Nurse Practitioner Project, patients' opinions were also sought about the impact of the nurse practitioner on their general practice (Stilwell *et al.*, 1987): 126 patients randomly selected from the practice age/sex register were asked a series of questions to find out if their perceptions of what the nurse practitioner did were accurate, if she was acceptable to patients in terms of their willingness to consult her and whether they felt it added to the services provided by the practice. Nearly three-quarters of the patients were able to describe one or more of the tasks performed by the nurse practitioner. A variety were mentioned including treating minor ailments, practical tasks, giving advice, preventative medicine, dealing with particular groups of the population such as the elderly, counselling and non-medical tasks. Her role was however first and foremost perceived as that of helping the doctor:

> *Housewife*: She helps the doctor by seeing patients that need advice or have not got a serious problem.

> *Male Factory Worker*: She takes care of the doctor's patients who have minor injuries and when the doctors are full she helps to see people.

Nevertheless, 10 per cent of patients felt that the nurse practitioner did much the same as the doctor and although there was a female doctor in the practice, the fact that the nurse practitioner was a woman was obviously important for some patients:

> *Female Nursery Nurse*: She sees people who would prefer to speak to a woman than a man.

Almost half the patients in the sample had already consulted the nurse practitioner and most of them had personally chosen to see her, that is they had not simply been referred to her by the doctor. Their reasons for doing so were various, for example because of the nature of the problem they had:

> *Housewife*: My children had German Measles, so we obviously didn't want to wait with other people, so we were allowed to go straight in after first phoning the surgery.

Or to save time:

> *Female Veterinary Assistant*: To be quite frank, because the waiting room was full.

Or because of the nurse practitioner's personal qualities:

> *Male Engineer*: Because she is more patient and understanding and has more time to listen than the doctor.

Although over half of these patients said they would be prepared to go back to the nurse practitioner again, it was apparent that for some patients the concept was not acceptable:

> *Male Nurse*: She is not medically trained and can't prescribe any medication.

> *Housewife*: I only go to the doctors when really necessary and it is important.

Whilst 18 per cent of patients did not hold strong views about the nurse practitioner, 41 per cent felt that the concept was a good one mainly because it improved the practice organization by being time-saving and more efficient.

> *Housewife*: It takes a considerable load off the doctor and eliminates waiting time in the surgery.

> *Male Retail Manager*: A nurse practitioner is an asset to the smooth running at the surgery and also an extra help to both doctor and patient.

However, of the patients, 40 per cent were opposed to the idea mainly because they felt the nurse practitioner lacked ability in clinical diagnosis:

> *Male Sales Manager*: I consider my problems and illnesses are for doctors to diagnose, I cannot see the point of having doctors if practitioners do the same job.

> *Housewife*: You go to see a doctor and a doctor you want to see.

Although, therefore, there is support for the development of the nurse practitioner role among both providers and consumers and existing evaluations of the role in practice demonstrate that nurses working in an extended way in general practice have much to offer, moves towards any formal recognition of the concept in this country are developing very slowly. The reasons for this are both complex and varied.

GP stances

Martin (1987) has identified four advantages of employing a practice nurse for the general practitioner:

> Flexibility. The practice nurse is based at the health centre and is available for tasks delegated by the general practitioner.

Financial benefit. Certain services, such as immunisations and cytotests carry a fee claimable from the family practitioner committee. The practice nurse can do these tasks for which the general practitioner may not have time.

Complex organisational, negotiation between the general practitioner and the nurse manager is removed.

Time saving . . . . The doctor has a number of time consuming tasks taken from him by the nurse who is usually more competent at performing them.

Although clearly practice nurses are of enormous benefit to a general practice, many doctors still do not employ a nurse in their surgery. Despite the recent increase in the number of practice nurses, compared to the number of general practitioners, their number is insufficient and varies by region ranging from 48 in the Mersey Regional Health Authority to 275 in the West Midlands Regional Health Authority (Bowling, 1987). The explanation lies in the fact that a number of GPs misunderstand the nature and skills of nurses. Others feel that in spite of the 70 per cent reimbursement scheme, to employ a practice nurse is too costly. Many surgeries simply do not have enough space to accommodate extra staff even if they wished to do so and some GPs are sceptical about the value of preventative medicine, an area where a practice nurse can be particularly useful. Even among those GPs who do employ a practice nurse there are fears that if nurses are allowed to extend their role to assume some of the tasks hitherto performed by doctors, they may gradually erode the doctor's role leading to an increase in medical unemployment. This entrenched attitude on the part of GPs is borne out by the opinions of the 300 practice nurses interviewed in the West Midlands (Greenfield *et al.*, 1987): 15 per cent of these nurses felt that the GP's attitude was the factor which prevented them from extending their own role further and 46.4 per cent felt that this was the major barrier which limited practice nurses in general.

Nurse aspirations

The US experience and the two experiments which have taken place in the UK (Reedy *et al.*, 1980c; Stilwell *et al.*, 1987) tend to suggest that doctors' fears are groundless. Only one of the trainee physician's assistants' colleagues said she felt insecure and hostile to him and she missed the initial briefing during which his role was explained. During the Birmingham Nurse Practitioner Project other members of the primary health care team, GPs, nurses and clerical staff were asked for their views about extending the role of the nurse in general practice. The nurses and GPs supported the development of this role although one said that he felt the skills of a nurse practitioner were more appropriately suited to preventative medicine:

GP: I should like to see the nurse practitioner take a less active role in curative medicine and instead take a more positive role in preventive work, such as seeking out problems in the community before they reach a crisis, improving the immune status of the practice, health education and monitoring patients with diseases that need to be reviewed regularly. Lack of having to make many clinical decisions in previous experience may lead to wrong clinical judgements being made, though we are all susceptible to making wrong clinical judgements. The bias towards curative medicine may reflect such a bias in nurse training as indeed it occurs also in medical training.

The clerical staff too expressed their satisfaction:

Practice Manager: She is able to see and advise a patient with any kind of medical matter and also is able to spend time with patients and is able to make one feel at ease.

Receptionist: It takes the workload off the doctors for minor ailments.

Receptionist: It helps patients, particularly young mums who sometimes need reassurance on relatively minor matters, also women who prefer to talk to a woman about gynaecological problems. It also helps the receptionist having a qualified person to refer to if the doctor is busy.

Although evidence does suggest that there is support among members of the RCN for developing the nurse practitioner role (RCN, 1987) and among practice nurses in the West Midlands (Greenfield *et al.*, 1987) whose views it is reasonable to expect are fairly representative, only 15 per cent wished to extend their role further and many nurses are ambivalent about the desirability of this. Some felt that if their role was extended to encompass a range of medical tasks they would be obliged to move away from the traditional style of caring. Others were frightened by the idea of having to perform delegated tasks for which they felt they have not received adequate training and by the possible legal consequences resulting from mismanagement of patients' problems.

The two issues of appropriate training and the legal position of the nurse are central to the debate. Although the Cumberledge Report (DHSS, 1986) recommended the introduction of a nurse practitioner it did not clearly specify what the appropriate qualification should be nor the tasks for which a nurse practitioner would qualify.

Jeffree (1988) suggests six sources of continuing education for the practice nurse:

• support a local practice nurse group
• organize practice meetings, with other members of the practice team, to discuss clinical issues and practice procedures and protocol
• attend conferences

- attend study days
- attend refresher courses
- read journals, books and papers.

However, it is undoubtedly a difficult – if not impossible – area for nurses. Although the first recognized course for practice nurses was approved by the English National Board in 1985, at present practice nurse courses are still few and far between and the study by Greenfield *et al.* (1987) also suggested that even where courses do exist the opportunities for nurses to participate in them may be limited due to the unwillingness of the GP to permit them to have the required time off to attend. Out of the 300 nurses interviewed, only half had been on an in-service training course whilst in their present post (44 per cent had been in the post for more than five years) yet 69 per cent of nurses thought their role was already extended beyond what they had been taught in their basic training. Furthermore, it may be that this is a group which has a particular need for continuing education since studies which have examined the social characteristics of practice nurses (Reedy *et al.*, 1980a; Greenfield *et al.*, 1987) have shown that most are aged between 30 and 45 years and are married with children. For many women practice nursing was the way in which they resumed work after a careeer break devoted to raising their families.

Conclusions

If practice nurses are already taking on a role for which they have been unprepared in their general training, it is not surprising that many of them are doubtful about the advisability of widening their range of tasks still further. An additional factor is the uncertainty about the legal position of nurses in general practice.

Here there are two main areas of legal responsibility to be taken into consideration. It appears that if a nurse is carrying out an activity which is a nursing responsibility for which she has received formal training, then she will be liable under her own professional ethics. If on the other hand she is performing a task which falls outside these routine nursing duties she is only liable if it can be proved that she has been adequately trained. The nurse's legal position when performing delegated tasks is therefore far from clear-cut. Although it is clearly a waste of medical manpower for doctors to perform tasks which an appropriately trained nurse could carry out equally well, until the twin problems of training and legal status have been addressed and resolved, it is hard to envisage that the introduction of a formally recognized nurse practitioner role into UK general practice will be speedily implemented.

References

Bowling, A. (1981) *Delegation in General Practice – A Study of Doctors and Nurses.* London: Tavistock Publications.

Bowling, A. (1987) The future role. *Nursing Times* (April 29), **83**(17), 31–3.

Cartwright, A. and Scott, R. (1961) The work of a nurse employed in a general practice. *British Medical Journal*, **1**, 807–13.

Cartwright, A. and Anderson, R. (1981) *General Practice Revisited.* London: Tavistock Publications.

Consumers Association (1987) Making your doctor better. *Which?* (May), 230–3.

Department of Health and Social Security (1986) *Neighbourhood Nursing – A Focus for Care.* Report of the Community Nursing Review, 32. London: HMSO.

Department of Health and Social Security (1987) *Health Services Development. Community Nursing Services and Primary Health Care Teams*, HC (87) 29: HC(FP) (87) 10. London: DHSS.

Greenfield, S., Stilwell, B. and Drury, M. (1987) Practice nurses: Social and occupational characteristics. *Journal of the Royal College of General Practitioners*, **37**, 341–5.

Jeffree, P. (1988) The practice nurse's role, past, present and future. *The Practice Nurse*, **1**(3), 106–7.

Jesop, M. (1986) Most practice nurses are not nurse practitioners. *General Practitioner* (31 October), 20.

Marplan Limited (1985) *NHS Nurses.* Report conducted for NHS (8 August 1985). London: Marplan.

Martin, C. (1987) Practice makes perfect. *Nursing Times* (29 April), **83**(17), 28–30.

Ramsay, J., McKenzie, J. and Fish, D. (1982) Physicians and nurse practitioners: do they provide equal health care? *American Journal of Public Health*, **72**, 55–7.

Reedy, B.L. (1978) *The New Health Practitioners in America: A Comparative Study.* London: King Edward's Hospital Fund for London and Pitman Medical Publishing.

Reedy, B.L., Metcalfe, A.V., de Roumarie, M. and Newell, D.J. (1980a) The social and occupational characteristics of attached and employed nurses in general practice. *Journal of the Royal College of General Practitioners*, **30**, 471–82.

Reedy, B.L., Metcalfe, A.V., de Roumarie, M. and Newell, D.J. (1980b) A comparison of the activities and opinions of attached and employed nurses in general practice. *Journal of the Royal College of General Practitioners*, **30**, 483–9.

Reedy, B.L., Steward, T.I. and Quick, J.B. (1980c) Attachment of a physician's assistant to an English general practice. *Journal of the Royal College of General Practitioners*, **230**, 665–6.

Royal College of General Practitioners and Office of Population Censuses and Surveys (1981) *Morbidity Statistics from General Practice. Diagnostic Classification Reference Manual.* Titchfield: RCGP/OPCS.

Royal College of Nursing (1987) *Response to the Consultation on Primary Health Care Initiated by the Department of Health and Social Security.* London: RCN.

Secretaries of State for Social Services, Wales, Northern Ireland and Scotland (1986) *Primary Health Care – An Agenda for Discussion.* London: HMSO.

Secretaries of State for Social Services, Wales, Northern Ireland and Scotland (1987) *Promoting Better Health. The Government's Programme for Improving Primary Health Care.* London: HMSO.

Spitzer, W.O., Sackett, D.L. and Sibley, J.C. (1974) The Burlington randomised trial of the nurse practitioner. *New England Journal of Medicine*, **290**, 251–6.

Stilwell, B. (1985) GP's have 'nothing to fear' from the nurse practitioner. *Pulse*, (June 15), 28.

Stilwell, B., Greenfield, S., Drury, M. and Hull, F. (1987) A nurse practitioner in general practice: working style and pattern of consultations. *Journal of the Royal College of General Practitioners*, **37**, 154–7.

Watkins, L. and Wagner, E. (1982) Nurse practitioner and physician adherence to standing orders criteria for consultation or referral. *American Journal of Public Health*, **72**, 22–9.

Evolution in Community Care: The Role of the Community Pharmacist

Alison Blenkinsopp

What role for the community pharmacist?

'What is the future for general practice pharmacists?' Such was the question posed by Dr Gerard Vaughan, then Minister for Health, in his opening speech to the British Pharmaceutical Conference in 1981 (Vaughan, 1981). 'One knows there is a future for hospital and for industrial pharmacists', Dr Vaughan assured his audience, 'but there was no identified role for the general practice [community] pharmacist', he said. Commenting that pharmacists enjoyed the public's trust but were unable to make full use of the potential of their skills, Dr Vaughan argued that change must come from the profession itself. 'It is for pharmacists' he said, 'to work out their destiny and for the government to tell them whether it is legally, parliamentarily and financially possible.'

That statement followed an earlier announcement that a 'wide-ranging' inquiry into the system by which pharmacists were paid by the NHS was to be conducted. The government-sponsored Nuffield Inquiry into pharmacy began in 1983 and sought to define the pharmacist's future role. Publication of the Inquiry's findings in 1986 (Nuffield Foundation, 1986) was followed by the Government's White Paper *Promoting Better Health* in November 1987, setting out future policy for primary health care in the community. Fortunately for the pharmacy profession, both the Nuffield Inquiry Report and *Promoting Better Health* supported a developed role for the community pharmacist in an era where the professions had been increasingly and visibly threatened by outside pressures. The past decade had seen not only the monopolies of solicitors and opticians challenged but also the clinical freedom of doctors curtailed with the introduction of a

'Limited List' for National Health Service (NHS) prescribing. In contrast to these changes it was proposed in the Nuffield Inquiry Report and endorsed by the Government that the community pharmacist should take on new responsibilities in an 'extended role'.

A historical perspective

Pharmacy has been termed a marginal or quasi-profession (Denzin and Mettlin, 1986: McCormack, 1956) because of its failure to control the reason for its existence, that is, while the responsibility for prescribing drugs has always remained firmly within the domain of the medical profession, the pharmacist has been restricted to dispensing of medicines. Even this process has not remained exclusively the province of the pharmacist, and disputes about the rights of doctors and pharmacists to dispense prescriptions in rural areas remain to the present day.

In the pre-NHS period, community pharmacists dispensed relatively fewer prescriptions than today and had more time to act as advisers to those members of the public who did not consult the doctor for financial and other reasons. A visit to the local 'chemist' for free advice and the purchase of remedies over the counter was for many people an alternative to the more expensive physician and his drugs.

The inception of the NHS in 1948 brought about financial and professional security for community pharmacists, with expectations of increased numbers of prescriptions giving financial security. Such expectations were fulfilled, but the steady closure of pharmacy businesses during the next decades resulted in a dwindling number of community pharmacies dealing with an inexorably rising number of prescriptions and a vastly increased dispensing workload. It was not difficult, then, to predict that the community pharmacist was likely to become a dispenser of medicines rather than of advice, given the new circumstances and time constraints. The burgeoning pharmaceutical industry, with its increasingly sophisticated and elegantly-formulated drugs, gradually made the pharmacist's traditional manufacturing and compounding role redundant. Today, only a minority of prescriptions require the pharmacist to physically manufacture a medicine; for the most part pre-prepared products are labelled and dispensed. Little wonder, then, that the Minister of Health might express uncertainty at the role which the community pharmacist had to play in primary health care, and that he might question the future of this branch of the profession.

The Nuffield Inquiry

It was against this background, in 1981, that the Government announced that a major review of pharmacy practice was to be carried out. The Nuffield Inquiry was set up in 1983 and was funded by the Government to examine all aspects of pharmacy practice. The Committee of Inquiry consisted of 13 members, six of whom were pharmacists, three doctors, and four from other backgrounds outside the health care professions. A call for evidence from interested organizations and individuals was issued in 1984, and after sifting through a vast amount of data, the Inquiry published its report in March 1986.

The Nuffield Report was welcomed by pharmacy as a 'positive and independent' confirmation that not only was there a role for the community pharmacist, but that newer, exciting areas of practice were envisaged. Manna from heaven indeed to those pharmacists who had feared that the Inquiry might recommend unpalatable measures or suggest that community pharmacists were over-qualified for the job which they did. The new term 'extended role' became part of the vocabulary of pharmacy, promising developments in community pharmacy practice including visits by pharmacists to housebound patients at home and to residential and nursing homes to act as a medicines adviser, closer collaboration with general medical practitioners (GPs) in the prescribing of drugs and the reporting of adverse reactions to drugs. The Nuffield Report re-emphasized the traditional advisory role of the pharmacist on minor symptoms, and pronounced that the developing area of health promotion was one where community pharmacists had a contribution to make.

However, the fundamental thrust of the Nuffield Report was not that these duties and responsibilities should be additional to the pharmacist's dispensing function; rather that pharmacists must delegate some responsibility to other members of staff in order that time be generated for the 'extended role'. The Nuffield Report commented that 'The dispensing of many prescriptions could be shown, after the event, not to have required the personal attention of the pharmacist'. Looking to the future, and an increasing use of information technology in primary health care, Nuffield saw the developing sophistication of pharmacy computer systems and patient medication records and concluded that the pharmacist need not directly supervise the dispensing of each prescription. Recommending that the Council of the Pharmaceutical Society give careful consideration to the degree of supervision needed, the Nuffield Report stressed that the degree to which any pharmacist wished to delegate responsibility should be decided by that individual pharmacist.

Pharmacy's response to Nuffield. The 96 recommendations contained in the Nuffield Report were debated at length by the Council of the Royal Pharmaceutical Society of Great Britain, the body responsible for leading the profession into any 'new' role, and for the initiation and implementation of change. Consultation with the profession was achieved by a series of meetings where local pharmacists could make their views felt to visiting members of Council.

As far as delegation of professional responsibility for dispensing was concerned, fewer than half of the 190 local branches submitted any comment on their views. Of those who did so, some two-thirds were opposed to any delegation during the dispensing process. Thus, while the concept of an 'extended role' was generally accepted, the prospect of any change in the dispensary was apparently viewed with deep suspicion. Council considered the views expressed during the consultation process and decided that for development of professional practice in community pharmacy, changes must be made in the requirements for supervision of dispensing by the pharmacist. Rather than being required by law to directly supervise the dispensing process, Council sought to create a professional requirement that the pharmacist should see each prescription 'at some stage' during dispensing. The stage at which the prescription was seen or checked would be left to the pharmacist's professional discretion. This view was substantially less radical than Nuffield's original suggestion that the pharmacist need not see some prescriptions at all. Council policy was also that any delegation could only be to trained technicians, and that each pharmacy must have a written procedure and policy for such delegation to take place.

The Government's view. Promoting Better Health, the long-awaited White Paper defining future policy for primary health care endorsed many of the recommendations of the Nuffield Report. The theme of delegation of responsibility for supervision of dispensing was taken up in the White Paper, which stated clearly that dispensing technicians should be given greater responsibility in order to free the pharmacist's time and facilitate new roles and services. Specific roles were identified in the White Paper for community pharmacists, with remuneration. These were the keeping of patient medication records for elderly and confused patients, and the provision of pharmaceutical services to residential homes. Funding was promised 'at an appropriate time' to develop the pharmacist's role in health promotion and to fund research into pharmacy practice.

Implementation of the Nuffield recommendations. Fierce debate within the profession on the issue of supervision of dispensing has raged within the columns of the pharmaceutical press since publication of the Nuffield Report in 1986 and the Royal Pharmaceutical Society's Council's consultative document on policy in 1987. Some pharmacists were concerned that if some dispensing tasks were delegated to technicians then there might no longer be a need for pharmacists at all. Others argued that their less ethically-minded pharmacist colleagues would abuse any new system and absent themselves from their pharmacy. Pharmacists expressed concern about the major change proposed to their professional role and their uncertainties about the future were understandable.

The Society's Council reiterated its policy on supervision in June 1988 (Ferguson, 1988) despite pressure for a policy U-turn applied both within and outside Council itself. There has been intense speculation about the 'true' views of community pharmacists about the issue. An unofficial 'referendum' in May 1988 found more than 80 per cent of respondents to be opposed to any change in supervision requirements, but the referendum achieved only a 5 per cent response rate. By September 1988 plans were being made for a Special General Meeting of the Royal Pharmaceutical Society, at which Council's opponents intended to bring a motion of 'No Confidence' in the Council over the supervision issue. By this time the argument had been honed down to one point of issue, namely whether the pharmacist should check every prescription at the final stage, just before handing the finished product to the patient. Council's view was that the pharmacist should exercise his or her professional judgement about the need for a final check. Such a check is not currently a legal requirement.

The Special General Meeting was held in April 1989 and resulted in a narrow but clear majority (371 to 306) for a motion of no confidence in the Council. The issue that brought about this unprecedented event was the exclusion from the proposed model procedure of the 'final check' by a qualified pharmacist. As a result the Council set up a working party on the issue to report within three months. In October 1989 the Council agreed unanimously to retain 'the final check' after receiving legal opinion that their action fell within the meaning of current legislation. The way was therefore clear for the Society to seek to expand the domain of professional tasks in the manner suggested by the Nuffield Report (*Pharmaceutical Journal*, 1989c).

The role of dispensing technicians

Relatively small numbers of community pharmacists currently employ trained dispensing technicians, i.e. those who have undergone a recognized training programme leading to a certificate of qualification. The Nuffield Inquiry considered the role of the dispensing technician to be fundamental to that of the community pharmacist and proposed that more responsibility should be given to trained technicians. The changes in the requirement for supervision and development of the extended role envisaged by Nuffield were seen by the Committee of Inquiry to be feasible only by greater use of trained technicians.

The situation in hospital pharmacy is in marked contrast to that in community pharmacy. The utilization of trained support staff is universal in hospital pharmacy; technicians are employed in all hospital pharmacy departments and some technicians already have a role which is extended from the traditional.

Should community pharmacists wish to pursue the implementation of the Nuffield recommendations the need to employ greater numbers of trained technicians is self-evident because there are still community pharmacists who carry out the mechanics of dispensing themselves when that part of the process can readily be delegated to a trained member of pharmacy staff. Over the next decade the proportion of community pharmacies which employs trained dispensing staff will undoubtedly increase. The wider utilization of support staff in community pharmacies can only be of benefit to patients because it will allow pharmacists to spend more time talking to their customers and patients and giving more information about medicines and health.

The community pharmacist's role outside the pharmacy

The extended role of the pharmacist includes the provision of services to residential and nursing homes. Community pharmacists will be paid to make regular visits to local homes and give advice and training on the safe storage and administration of medicines. Some community pharmacists are already providing a service of this kind but pharmacists' involvement in services to residential and nursing homes is increasing so that rather than simply providing a dispensing service the pharmacist will train non-medical staff in the homes and give advice on working systems to ensure that the residents in the homes get the correct prescribed medicine at the right time. Policies for medicines storage and administration to patients are under development to cover local districts and ensure consistency and high standards in all homes. This development of the pharmacist's role and completion of a training package will be a prerequisite to providing the service.

Another suggested development of the community pharmacist's role is in domiciliary visits – visits to patients in their own homes. Many patients are housebound and thus unable to visit the pharmacy to collect a prescription or buy medicines and the proportion of such patients is likely to increase with demographic change and greater numbers of elderly people in the community. A large number of community pharmacists already provide a limited prescription delivery service but the concept of domiciliary visits implies that the pharmacist would spend time with the patient discussing his or her medication, explaining about the correct use and storage of medicines and dealing with any problems encountered by the patient.

Currently there is a major obstacle to community pharmacists leaving their shop premises other than for very brief periods because the law requires their presence to supervise the dispensing of prescriptions and sale of certain medicines. Even the proposed changes in supervision requirements are not intended to allow the pharmacist to leave the pharmacy for long periods. Consequently for the development of services such as those to residential homes and domiciliary visits within working hours the community pharmacist will inevitably have to employ another pharmacist to provide professional cover. Suggestions for achieving role development include alterations in pharmacy opening hours and the employment of part-time pharmacists for a few hours a week.

Community services pharmacists – what is their role?

The post of Community Services Pharmacist (CSP) was created to bridge the gap between hospital and community care. Community Services Pharmacists are employed by the NHS via the hospital pharmacy service and their numbers have been increasing steadily over the last decade. The role of the CSP has not yet been fully defined and this branch of the pharmacy profession is at an early stage in its development. Generally the CSP's role is seen as a coordinating one in the community, for example in ensuring consistency in medicines policies in the residential and nursing homes across an NHS district. Relationships between CSPs and community pharmacists appear to be variable and CSPs themselves have a wide variety of job descriptions and responsibilities. Antagonism towards CSPs is already detectable in some quarters from community pharmacists who are suspicious about the concept of the CSP and see this new pharmacist as a potential usurper of their role. CSPs themselves are currently trying to establish their professional territory and related specialist area (Taylor, 1988) and have been successful at creating a high profile both within and outside the profession.

Patient medication record

The White Paper *Promoting Better Health* promised funding for community pharmacists who kept records of medicines supplied to elderly and 'confused' patients. A small minority of pharmacists has been maintaining such records for some time and the benefits to patient care of record-keeping by the pharmacist have been demonstrated (Poston and Shulman, 1984). Benefits include detection of potential interactions between prescribed medicines, unintended high doses of medicines and potential interactions with medicines purchased over the counter. Records were kept manually by those pharmacists who kept them but several computer-based packages are now available and computerized records will probably become the norm. However, since patients are not required to register with one community pharmacist, in contrast to the situation with general medical practitioners, it is recognized that pharmacy-based records might be incomplete because patients may have their prescription dispensed at any pharmacy they choose. No one pharmacy would have a complete record of all prescriptions dispensed and medicines purchased by the patient.

The development of a patient-held computerized record to hold all medical information, details of prescribed medicines and those purchased over the counter could be a step forward. Trials of such record in the form of a SMART card (a plastic card with a magnetic strip containing information) are currently being conducted. All doctors' surgeries and community pharmacies in the area are equipped with a card reader and a computer which can write new information onto the card. Patient registration with pharmacies appears unlikely in the foreseeable future because of the limitations it would impose on the consumer's choice and a patient-held record seems to be a workable solution to the problem.

Original pack dispensing

The dispensing process currently involves the transfer of medicines from one pack to another because medicines are bought in bulk by the pharmacist and dispensed in smaller quantities. In such a transfer, there is always the possibility of error – tablet bottles being mixed up where there are several medicines on a prescription, for example. During the next few years a major change in dispensing will occur with the introduction of Original Pack Dispensing (OPD) where manufacturers will produce medicines in unit packs, each for a course of treatment. Medicines will be available in separate packs which will provide, say, one month's treatment. The dispensing process will therefore involve selecting the appropriate pack and labelling directly onto the original pack itself. The possibility of error will be reduced because the identity of the medicine will be clearly printed on the pack.

When OPD is introduced each pack of medicines will contain a leaflet to provide patients with more information about the medicines they are taking. The contents of the leaflets are under discussion but basic facts are likely to include what the medicine is used for, how to take it and any likely side effects. The supply of more information to patients about their medicines has been welcomed by patient and consumer groups. It is likely that community pharmacists will be increasingly asked for information by patients who have read the leaflets about their medication.

The impact of information technology on the practice of community pharmacy

Pharmacy is the most highly computerized of all the health professions; some 80% of community pharmacies have a computer system. The installation of such systems was initially prompted by the introduction of a professional requirement in 1985 that all medicine labels should be typed or mechanically printed. The requirement was initiated by the Society's Council and was greeted at the time with a mixed response from the profession because of the expense of purchasing a computer system (not reimbursable through the health service). Undoubtedly though, the Council's action spurred the development of computerized pharmacy systems and their widespread uptake.

The potential impact of information technology in the future is huge for pharmacy. There are now systems which incorporate complex labelling capabilities including facilities to identify drug interactions and keep full records of medicines purchased for minor ailments as well as those prescribed by the general practitioner. In the future it is likely that patient-held medical and medication records will become more widespread;

pharmacies will have card readers linked to their computer systems and may well have direct links to the computer in the local medical practice with access to information. Other developments include the availability of databases so that pharmacists will be able to access the latest information about medicines and treatment.

Links between community pharmacists and general practitioners

The Nuffield Inquiry Report identified the unsatisfactory working relationships which exist between many community pharmacists and GPs, saying 'At present contacts between pharmacist and GP mainly take place after a prescription has been made, on the initiative of the pharmacist, in circumstances likely to put the GP on the defensive' (Nuffield Foundation, 1986). The reference was to those occasions when pharmacists need to contact a prescriber to check a prescription because of an omission or possible error. Unfortunately such conversations form the majority of contacts between many pharmacists and doctors and do not promote a collaborative working relationship. Traditional professional boundaries and territoriality in addition to the geographical isolation of pharmacists and doctors have militated against the development of closer working.

The Nuffield Inquiry recommended that a system should be devised such that pharmacists and GPs would meet regularly to discuss matters of mutual interest, particularly ways of making prescribing more effective and less costly. This concept was supported by the White Paper *Promoting Better Health* and has led to the concept of Local Liaison Groups. A Local Liaison Group consists of community pharmacists and GPs who serve the same cohort of patients. These groups are in the very early stages of development and research will document their nature and effectiveness. More constructive and regular discussions between pharmacists and GPs should improve working relationships and benefit patients through sharing of information and rationalization of prescribing.

Health promotion

The involvement of community pharmacists in supplying information and advice on health education should be an appropriate development from their background of health knowledge. Since 1986 a national scheme for the distribution of health education leaflets has been in operation with leaflets being sent to every community pharmacy in the country. Attention is now being focussed on pharmacists' training in health issues with a view to introducing the subject in the undergraduate course and providing continuing education for those pharmacists already practising. Such training will be essential if pharmacists are to supplement the supply of written information with appropriate advice on modification of lifestyle and behaviour to improve health chances.

Treatment of minor illness

Traditionally the community pharmacist has been a source of advice on minor illness and this role was supported by both the Nuffield Inquiry Report and the White Paper *Promoting Better Health*. Research has shown that members of the public use self-medication for many of their symptoms and that they readily seek the pharmacist's advice (Office of Population Census and Survey, 1982; Cunningham-Burley and Maclean, 1987). The profession has been keen to encourage requests for advice from members of the public, indeed, since 1983 a national advertising campaign has been run by the National Pharmaceutical Association (the trade association of community pharmacists) with the slogan 'Ask your pharmacist, you'll be taking good advice'.

For pharmacists to provide an effective advisory service and refer patients to their doctor where a more serious condition is suspected, a sound training is required. Consumer studies have examined the quality and content of advice given by community pharmacists and have identified specific areas where improvements could be made in questioning skills and identification of potentially serious symptoms (Consumer Association, 1985; Anon, 1988). The involvement of pharmacy counter staff in the giving of advice was found to be high in these studies and the quality of advice given by assistants to be unacceptably low.

The Nuffield Inquiry, while supporting the pharmacist's role in advising about patients' symptoms said, 'we consider it important that the pharmacist should be properly educated and trained to perform this role which includes the ability to assess when an inquirer should be recommended to seek medical advice' (Nuffield Foundation, 1986). In the past little attention was paid to this area of practice in the pharmacy undergraduate course but the subject is now included in the curriculum of most schools of pharmacy and its importance in continuing education has been recognized, although further developments are still needed. Pharmacy counter staff are known to receive little or no training in advising about symptoms and the profession has recognized the need to develop training programmes for assistants.

Community pharmacy – which way forward?

The community pharmacist's original role as a compounder and dispenser of medicines has changed substantially during the last decades. Community pharmacists are considered by some to have undergone de-skilling and a reduction in their defined professional role. Pharmacy has now been given the opportunity to develop its role and functions with new areas of professional practice to replace the outmoded emphasis on the mechanics of dispensing. The increasing development of technology and the introduction of original pack dispensing will decrease still further the need for the pharmacist to be involved in the actual dispensing process other than in a checking capacity. The apparent reluctance of some members of the profession to accept the inevitability of change and to plan for the long-term future may jeopardize the rejuvenation of the community pharmacist's role in primary health care.

Community pharmacists have the chance to become more actively involved in promoting better health in the community by visiting patients and raising standards in the safe and effective use of medicines. The potential to maximize patient benefit from medication while minimizing costs exists through the channels of collaboration with doctors. Technology and the employment of trained support staff could free time for the pharmacist to devote more time to talking to customers. The provision of information and advice about medicines and health to the public could be vastly increased through the network of community pharmacies. With a Government which has stated in its White Paper on primary health care its intention that community pharmacists should delegate many of the tasks involved in dispensing in order to free time for other activities to the benefit of patients, it could be argued that if the profession is unable or unwilling to exact change, then the Government will do so. The events of the next few years may contribute to the development or the further de-skilling of community pharmacy practice.

References

Anonymous (1988) Over-the-counter advice. *Self-Health*, **18**, 4–8.
Cunningham-Burley, S. and Maclean, U. (1987) The role of the chemist in primary health care for children with minor complaints. *Social Science Medicine*, **24**, 371–7.
Consumers Association (1985) Advice across the chemist's counter. *Which?* 351–4.
Denzin, N.K. and Mettlin, C.J. (1986) Incomplete professionalisation: the case of pharmacy. *Social Forces*, **46**, 375–81.
Department of Health and Social Security (1987) *Promoting Better Health*. London: HMSO.
Ferguson, J. (1988) Supervision of dispensing. *Pharmaceutical Journal*, **240**, 772–3.
McCormack, T.H. (1956) The druggist's dilemma: Problems of a marginal occupation. *American Journal of Sociology*, **61**, 308–38.
Nuffield Foundation (1986) *Pharmacy. A Report to the Nuffield Foundation*. London: Nuffield Foundation.
Office of Population Census and Survey (1982) *Access to Primary Health Care*. London: HMSO.
Pharmaceutical Journal (1988a) Report on Council Meeting, **241**, June, 212–16.
Pharmaceutical Journal (1988b) Report 'Special General Meeting a Near Certainty', **241**, September, 400–2.
Pharmaceutical Journal (1989a) Report on Special General Meeting, **242**, April, 438–44.
Pharmaceutical Journal (1989b) Report on Council Meeting, **242**, June, 716–18.
Pharmaceutical Journal (1989c) Report on Council Meeting, **242**, October, 495–96.

Poston, J.W. and Shulman, S. (1984) Patient medication records in community pharmacy. *Pharmaceutical Journal*, **234**, 442–3.

Royal Pharmaceutical Society (1987) Council's consultative document on the Nuffield Report (1987). *Pharmaceutical Journal*, **238**, N1–N15.

Taylor, E. (reported) (1988) Hospital to community – bridging the gap. *Pharmaceutical Journal*, **241**, 400–2.

Vaughan, G. (reported) (1981) What future for general practice pharmacists? *Pharmaceutical Journal*, **227**, 300–1.

8 | The Diffusion of Innovation in Clinical Equipment

Brian Shaw

Introduction

The subject of technological innovation in medicine is inextricably bound up with the history of the medical profession. Equally the process of invention and implementation has taken the profession into collaboration with natural scientists and engineers (Reiser and Anbar, 1984). Over this century their collaborators have increasingly been located in manufacturing industry and a symbiotic relationship has grown up between medical consultants and industrial designers in medical equipment innovation. This chapter focusses on the process by which this relationship operates to bring about innovations in clinical equipment. It is based on an empirical study carried out by the author. This process was identified by the author through a survey of the development of 34 such innovations involving 11 manufacturing companies (Shaw, 1986). These innovations are enumerated in Table 8.1 in which an evaluation of contributions to clinical practice is attempted by the author on the basis of user opinions.

Two characteristics of the process were isolated as determining the power nexus and negotiating patterns associated with the introduction of a novel technology:

1 That any equipment that is to be potentially introduced into clinical use first needs clinical assessment and trial.
2 That 'state-of-the-art' clinical and diagnostic knowledge resides in the 'user', that is the consultant who thereby becomes gatekeeper to subsequent markets.

Table 8.1 Sample composition

Component	Basic innovation	Major improvement innovation	Minor improvement innovation	Failure	Total
1 Electrocardiograph		X			
2 Neonatal oxygen monitoring system	X				
3 Venous oxygen monitoring system	X				
4 Care system for casualty work			X		
5 Miniaturization of radiography equipment			X		
6 Topical magnetic resonance spectroscopy	X				
7 ECG recorder			X		
8 EEG recorder		X			
9 Multiple detector head gamma counter for radioimmunoassay			X		
10 Portable autoclave		X			
11 Autoclave for sterilization of sealed fluids		X			
12 Portable chart recorder		X			
13 Hot air sterilizer			X		
14 Radio pill telemetry system		X			
15 Cardiac monitor			X		
16 EEG wave analyser				X	
17 Safety tester			X		
18 Oxytocin infusion system	X				
19 Powered syringe driver with patient-operated demand system	X				
20 Portable battery operated variable speed syringe driver	X				
21 Fixed-speed syringe driver				X	
22 Continuous syringe driver with boost facility			X		
23 Respiratory recording and monitoring system	X				
24 Infusion pump			X		
25 Foetal monitoring/Oxytocin pump combination			X		
26 Wright peak flow meter	X				
27 Mini-Wright peak flow meter		X			

Table 8.1 continued

Component	Basic innovation	Major improvement innovation	Minor improvement innovation	Failure	Total
28 Perkins hand-held applanation tonometer		X			
29 Transfer test apparatus	X				
30 Exercise test monitor	X				
31 Oxylog				X	
32 Nasal airway resistance tester				X	
33 Mass spectrometer				X	
34 Anaesthesia equipment			X		
Totals	10	8	11	5	34

The user is the term used to embrace the system in the UK of 'centres of excellence' (the 15 undergraduate, 6 postgraduate teaching and research hospitals and 20 universities with hospital schools) having technicians, scientists, engineers, physicians and clinicians all working together to find new means of achieving better patient care through equipment innovations. The clinician, usually a 'consultant', specifies a need, for example a faster, more hygienic way of achieving a particular therapy. The scientist, engineers and technicians then work together with the consultant in an attempt to test out the conceptual basis of the solution to the need, usually in the form of a rough handmade prototype. Further development normally results in the other actors in the innovation process joining the team, i.e. the 'intermediaries' and the manufacturers.

Communication patterns

Because the means of carrying out and the results of the clinical trials are only immediately available to those who have done the trials, some means of dissemination of data to other potential users, intermediaries and manufacturers must be effected. The communication pattern in the sample was:

1 Personal contact though the worldwide networking system available to the researchers and clinicians in the UK.
2 Presentation of papers at international conferences, professional meetings and/or industrial liaison groups.
3 Publication of articles in professional journals.
4 Publication of books.
5 Presentation at international exhibitions.
6 DHSS circulars in *Health Equipment Information* (HEI).

Table 8.2 Communication patterns

	Basic	Major	Minor	Failures	Total
Personal contact	10	8	6	5	29
Presentation of papers	8	4	3	0	15
Journal articles	7	3	4	1	15
Books	2	0	0	0	2
International exhibitions	2	0	2	0	4
DHSS circulars	0	0	0	0	0
NRDC	0	0	1	0	1
Salesmen	0	2	2	1	5
Totals	29	17	18	7	71

7 British Technology Group licensing list.
8 Manufacturers' salesmen.

The dominance of the personal contact and higher level of communication present at the Basic Innovation Stage illustrated in Table 8.2 reflects the high level of communication between scientists, engineers and clinicians within the very efficient worldwide informal and formal networking systems connecting medical centres of excellence. International conferences are centres for the initial negotiation by companies with the presenters of papers regarding involvement in their research and/or development. Similarly, the presenters of the papers negotiate with the industrial partners concerning advice and funding for research and development (R & D). The result of this networking is a very close community of researchers and practitioners be they scientists, engineers or clinicians, who are very knowledgeable of the worldwide research activity and practice being carried out in their area of interest.

This networking becomes more effective the narrower the degree of specialization among the consultants and biomedical engineers. The strong linkages to sources of technology and information external to their establishments available on universally orientated R & D projects overcome problems of translating across contrasting coding schemes. This obviates the need for the specialized role of technological gatekeeper (Allen, 1977). This finding supports the work of Tushman and Katz (1980) and confirms the sociometric results of Myers (1983) that informal preference networks such as the 'invisible colleges' described by Crane (1972) are likely to be primary in the communication of state-of-the-art information. The consultant's loyalty therefore tends to be split between his or her establishment and the 'invisible college', with his or her links to the sources of technology and information external to the centres of excellence being a major source of the consultant's power within each centre.

The hospitals outside the 'centres of excellence' tend to have a lower research and technology base, especially in terms of the quantity and quality of equipment available to them. The consultant or a member of his/her team, becomes both 'technological' and 'market gatekeepers' for these hospitals with the respect of the effective use and purchase of medical equipment. The significance of the consultant in this process confirms the impression of 'professional dominance' found by Freidson (1970) and Greer's (1984a) observations of economic leverage.

Gordon (1962) observed that the bifurcated authority in health care provision results in continual negotiating among power groups. Outcomes of this negotiation stem from the alternative means of leverage. In fact Saltman and Young (1981) concluded that in spite of recent challenges to physician's powers, the physician's control over the key sources of uncertainty within the hospital production process may well still generate sufficient resources to enable physicians to deflect any efforts to relax their decision-making grip. The economic leverage of the consultants in the UK is expressed in their (1) impact on the innovation process, (2) the quality of diagnosis, treatment and research, with its attendant resource attraction, and (3) their signature to the Area Board requisitions for technology.

The consultant's decision is based on his perception of the effectiveness of the equipment in improving diagnostic skill or enhancing therapeutic ability. The prime basis for this judgement is the clinical results achieved by using this equipment. The acceptance, in part, of the results is a function of who carried out the clinical test and the degree of involvement of personal contacts in the network in their validation. This 'peer group' behaviour extend to the purchase of medical equipment used for diagnosis and therapy outside the field of the consultant's specialism as 'he knows whom to talk to in the network who can give him a considered opinion he would accept'. Greer's (1984b) findings that technologies designed by individual physicians are reviewed, judged and typically approved by the collegium of medical practitioners is supported by this research. The 'peer group' behaviour mirrored that found by Coleman *et al.* (1966) and Peterson and McPhee (1973) in the USA.

Rogers and Shoemaker's (1971) general proposition was that individuals may be expected to be more receptive to innovations which are congruent with the values and interests they have acquired in the course of their professional socialization. However Greer (1984b) found that when the participation of physicians in actual technological decisions was documented, a more complex picture emerged. Differentiated physician roles in decision systems expressed a technological specialization within the medical profession as well as the growth of hospitals as dynamic large-scale organizations specializing in sophisticated technology. Traditional hospital concerns with clinical medicine are greatly complicated by the separable concerns with the management of institutional growth and development. Greer's research suggests that the 'peer group' buyer behaviour, expressed through the bifurcated authority structure, relies upon the amount and nature of the power behind the leverage that is available to each party involved in the negotiations. This leverage is expressed in the three decisions systems: the collegium of medical practitioners, the fiscal–managerial and the strategic–institutional decision systems. However, research into medical technology decision-making does not seem to have addressed decisions other than those concerned with the adoption and diffusion of medical technology. The research into the generation, development, marketing and diffusion of the 34 medical equipment innovations studied here, attempts to fill that gap.

Because of the need for clinical trials a special relationship is needed between the clinical advisory and trial team on the one hand, and the potential manufacturer of the equipment on the other. Sometimes assessment and trial require a very elaborate study of how a particular piece of equipment can be used and to what effect. It is important that a systematic attempt is made to clarify how the equipment or the principle it embodies will advance the clinical task it is meant to assist, because human life may be at risk. The greater the research input, the more the power might appear to lie with the user in which the 'state-of-the-art' clinical knowledge resides. Blume (1985) affirms this hypothesis when he suggests that innovation *for* the health care system and innovation *by* the health care system becomes unclear. What appears to be two distinct processes are more probably to be regarded as a single innovation process in which user and designer are bound together by research.

Output-embodied benefits

The output-embodied benefits are those arising from the output made possible through the availability and use of the equipment. For example, a piece of medical equipment is capable of achieving a particular clinical objective – the Exercise Test Monitor developed by P.K. Morgan Ltd can measure any procedure involving ventilating and cardiac responses to exercise, examination and assessment of pulmonary and cardiac disease, exercise-induced asthma and the response to chemotherapy and the study of athletic training. The achievement of this clinical objective, in turn, gives the clinician a greater understanding of the bodily functions, greater diagnostic ability and the basis of further research. The experience of testing and evaluating the equipment before it becomes commercially available also gives the clinician intellectual stimulation (Harries, 1981), a significant advantage both in terms of research expertise and practise in the implementation of the therapy or diagnosis developed. In addition, the worldwide diffusion of knowledge, best practice and social benefits through the 'invisible college' increases the status of the consultant in the college. The closer these benefits are to the 'state-of-the-art' advances, the greater the benefit to the clinician, and therefore the more involved the consultant will want to be in the innovation process. Where these benefits are not present, he or she will try not to get involved. In the sample, in fact, another major output-embodied benefit to consultants was profit from running their own business when businesses were set up by consultants to take economic advantage of their knowledge and understanding of their particular area of expertise.

The evidence of differing abilities to obtain output-embodied benefits, especially when the abilities differ significantly between the user and the manufacturer, suggests that some shift in the balance of benefit could be achieved if the manufacturer could keep more innovation-related benefits personally and allocate innovation-related costs to others, i.e. users, suppliers, intermediaries. The need to shift the balance of benefit is the more compelling when, as research by Mansfield *et al.* (1977), Tewksbury *et al.* (1980) and Nathan Associates (1978) found, firms' 'private' rates of return from innovation (net return to the innovation firm) are much lower than the 'social' rates of return from innovation (net return to the innovator plus net return to all other private parties – innovation users, suppliers, imitators, etc. – affected by the innovation). Thus potentially low 'private' rates of return may deter the manufacturer from developing innovations that give high 'social' returns. Tewksbury *et al.* (1980) found that three of his sample of 20 innovations had social returns of 27, 37 and 104 per cent, and private returns of 0, 9 and less than 0 per cent. The ability to shift the balance of innovation benefit seems to be a function of the power of the parties in the innovation network and their relationship.

To delineate the innovation benefits more comprehensively, a distinction is required between quantifiable benefits (such as profits from sales of medical equipment or patent licensing fees) and unquantifiable benefits (such as trust in the manufacturer developed, say, as a result of close cooperation in the innovation development), a reduction in the 'social distance'. The 'intermediary', i.e. the Medical Research Council, benefits from the efficient use of its funding and personnel and acts as an effective medium for the transfer of technology. The manufacturer's benefit is embodied in the sales and profits from this innovative medical equipment and the enhanced corporate image created by developing socially responsible products. To the extent that the user's benefits identified can be quantified, the very existence of the innovative medical equipment creates on-going social benefits throughout the life cycle of the equipment.

Source of identification of need

As illustrated in Table 8.3 the present study showed the incidence of identification of the need for the innovation by the medical user to be greater the nearer the innovation was to the basic equipment end of the innovation spectrum. Also (in 21 out of the 34 innovations) there was complete dominance by the users and intermediaries, in the identification of user need.

Table 8.3 Source of identification of need

Classification of innovations	Total	Identification of need					
		User		Manufacturer		Intermediary	
		No.	%	No.	%	No.	%
Basic	10	9	90%	0	0%	1	10%
Major	8	6	75%	1	12.5%	1	12.5%
Minor	10	7	70%	3	30%	0	0%
Failures	6	4	66%	1	17%	1	17%
Totals	34	26	76%	5	15%	3	9%

Users

The result of this user gain of output-embodied benefits was that in the sample of 34 innovations, 26 were developed through multiple and continuous user–intermediary–manufacturer interaction, 22 of these were successful, one being too early to judge and three being failures. The failures were due principally to the unsatisfactory technical performance of the equipment. A successful innovation was one that achieved the technical and commercial objectives set for it by the manufacturer. Although these objectives would tend to differ between different companies, especially the multi-nationals such as Picker International and the newly formed companies such as Innotron Ltd, adherence to the achievement of these objectives stimulated the companies to further involvement in new design.

The frequency with which the 'norm' of multiple and continuous user–intermediary–manufacturer interaction was displayed in the sample was significant, as shown in Table 8.4. As indicated, the interaction consisted not only of joint prototype development, testing, product evaluation and marketing but also joint prototype development and product marketing and joint product specification and marketing. The close interaction by the user with the manufacturer in the prototype development, testing and evaluation, marketing and joint specification on the 'basic' and 'major' improvements differed from that found by Gardiner and Rothwell (1985) where the user was principally involved in the re-innovation stage. This difference might be expected where 'state-of-the-art' clinical and diagnostic knowledge resides in the user, and the balance of output-embodied benefits can be gained by him or her. This knowledge ensured that the equipment being developed was designed to meet the clinical and/or diagnostic objectives set by the clinician. However, with only a minor increase in multiple user–manufacturer interaction, albeit not intense, commercial success was achievable.

Reclassifying the basic, major and minor innovations to 'user domi-

Table 8.4 Frequency of multiple and continuous user–manufacturer interaction by classification of innovation

Classification of innovations	No.	%	Form of user–manufacturer interaction					
			Joint testing, product evaluation and marketing		Joint prototype development and marketing		Joint product specification and marketing	
			No.	%	No.	%	No.	%
Basic equipment innovation	10	29%	10	100%	8	80%	8	80%
Major improvement innovation	8	24%	8	100%	6	75%	4	50%
Minor improvement innovation	10	29%	5	50%	3	30%	1	10%
Failures	6	18%	2	33%	2	33%	0	0%
Totals	34	100%	25	74%	19	56%	13	38%

Table 8.5 Frequency of user–dominated innovative processes and the degree of user–manufacturer interaction associated with the process

Classification of innovations	No.	%	Joint testing, product evaluation and marketing		Joint prototype development and marketing		Joint product specification and marketing	
			No.	%	No.	%	No.	%
User dominated	18	53%	17	94%	17	94%	13	72%
Manufacturer dominated	16	47%	8	50%	2	12%	0	0%
Totals	34	100%	25	74%	19	56%	13	38%

nated' and 'manufacturer dominated' (Von Hippel, 1977) and relating them to the degree of user–manufacturer interaction, the same pattern of user dominance emerged (Table 8.5). In 17 (94 per cent) of the 18 'user dominated' innovations (a user prototype was developed), after the transfer of the user innovations to the manufacturer, the user continued joint prototype development, testing, evaluation and marketing of their products with the manufacturer. In 13 cases the user specified the final product with the manufacturer. In eight of the 16 'manufacturer dominated' innovations, the user tested and evaluated the manufacturer's prototype and helped market the product. One user helped develop the prototype, test, evaluate and market it and one helped to develop the manufacturer's prototype and market the final product.

Intermediaries

Other important actors in the innovation process studied here are the intermediaries. These are the UK Medical Research Council (MRC), British Technology Group (BTG) (previously the National Research Development Council, NRDC), the Department of Health (DoH) consultants and the Department of Industry (DoI). The MRC scientists or engineers are seconded to units which do not have the necessary scientific or engineering skills in the support of the consultant or which invent and develop their own innovations with manufacturers. The BTG are responsible for patenting public sector innovations. They also have a specialist in medical equipment who acts as a link between the users, MRC and manufacturers. He advises manufacturers on user and MRC inventions and users and MRC on appropriate manufacturers to approach for possible collaboration. The DoH has a consultant in every medical discipline who links into the networking system and who enjoys, and is encouraged to have, good contacts with equipment manufacturers. These consultants act as a useful link between the manufacturers and the users primarily by placing the manufacturer's prototype into the appropriate medical centres for testing and evaluation. Once the entrée is effected there is no restriction by the DoH on any subsequent user–manufacturer interaction.

A registered UK medical equipment supplier can ask the DHSS to arrange for their expert to give a clinical and commercial view regarding equipment. The Department also advises on relevant international safety standards. The DoH also fund R & D and feasibility studies and prototype developments. The funding is initially for a feasibility study but if the new idea or product appears feasible, further funding will be made available for all stages up to the prototype stage. The normal level of funding is 50 per cent of the cost of development up to prototype stage. The department also has a pump-priming budget to seed new products and buy in larger numbers than required for evaluation purposes for distribution around the regions. The DoI has a system for the purchase of pre-production equipment.

The importance of these intermediaries can be seen in that within the sample the MRC acted as intermediaries for 12 of the innovations, the DoH for four and the DoI for one. The BTG patented 11 of the sample, of which 10 were successful. The smaller companies found this to be the major benefit of their interactions with the intermediaries in that the BTG's financial muscle and patent know-how could defend them from predators. The MRC, DoH and DoI together placed the prototypes of 13 innovations for testing and evaluation. The DoI arranged the placing of pre-production models of Innotron's 'Hydragamma-16' in nine radio-immunoassay laboratories in Cardiff, Glasgow, Birmingham, London, Amsterdam and Miami. The total testing time in these nine centres was approximately 1000 hours. A major stimulus given by the intermediaries was the initial purchase of 14 of the 34 innovations. In addition, MRC experts, such as Dr Wright, wrote papers about the Respiratory Recording and Monitoring System (Innovation 23) in the *Proceedings of the Physiological Society* and the *Third International Symposium on Ambulatory Monitoring*, the main means of communication with potential users. Another example was Dr Wright's paper in 1978 ('A miniature Wright peak flow meter', *British Medical Journal* 2). These writings stimulated interest in this equipment and gave credibility to the manufacturer thus helping to ensure its commercial success.

Manufacturers

The third actor in the innovation process is the manufacturer who is concerned with gaining added-value from the centres of excellence and users when creating, developing and marketing the 34 medical equipment innovations. The mechanisms used were as follows:

1 Appropriating user-knowledge to themselves.
2 Transferring costs to the user's intermediaries and suppliers.
3 Increasing private returns by gaining increased market penetration through cooperation with the users and intermediaries.
4 The coupling of 'outside' producer champions to 'inside' product champions.

Appropriation of user knowledge

This appropriation is illustrated by the development of the Exercise Test Monitor by P.K. Morgan Ltd. Mr Morgan, the Managing Director, noticed that Dr Cotes of the MRC Pneumoconiosis Research Unit had written a paper on the 'Tripartite Test' which quantified the effects of the exercise. He therefore initiated a period of intensive collaboration with Dr Cotes to develop equipment that could plot the necessary data in the form required.

The software programing for the system represented four years of high-quality work. The origin of this work was a BASIC programing system developed by Dr Nelson Braslow, a cardio-respiratory physician at Massachusetts General Hospital. The chief engineer of P.K. Morgan developed the MGH work by translating the BASIC into FORTRAN, COBOL and PASCAL programs. These provided the basis for comparison of data.

Knowing the output requirement of the Exercise Test Monitor, due to the close contacts with potential users, Mr Morgan was attracted by the unique method of mathematical analysis developed at the Respiratory Department of Guy's Hospital to scale and measure information about body plethysmography. Having checked the acceptability of this program to the system being developed by the company, Mr Morgan agreed with Guy's a right to use the program, to lock into their research in the respiratory field and to accept their consultancy help in incorporating the mathematical analysis into the company's equipment. The incorporation of this user knowledge in the monitor gave the company a major competitive lead.

Transferring costs to the user

R & D costs

In 20 of the innovations the essential characteristics of the product were identified at the concept stage, resulting in the R & D work addressing specific technological problems rather than operating across a broad general technological front. This reduced development time, enabled the manufacturers to delineate clearly the R & D needed and enabled the channelling of technological problems and focussing of activities. This in turn resulted in reduced development time and cost and more effective translation of user need into technological form.

Examples of the synergy gained in R & D were the concentration on clearly defined existing areas in 20 of the innovations, and synergy across other projects in nine cases. In fact a major use of R & D resources was in continuous redesign identified through interaction with and feedback from the users and competitive activity. Coupled with this redesign was the elimination of technical and engineering faults. These activities were present in the on-going development of 16 of the innovations. The manufacturers' R & D however, was supplemented by that of 13 major research and professional institutes. Detailed technical specifications and the nature of the base technology were given to the manufacturer by the medical user in 13 of the innovations.

The collaboration between the user, intermediaries and manufacturers created a situation where in 25 of the innovations, the manufacturers' engineers/scientists understood the user environment and identified the key variables in the user needs. The joint activities, i.e. joint prototype testing, evaluation and marketing in 25, the joint prototype development and marketing in 19 and joint product specification and marketing in 13 of the innovations, also determined a high level of 'technological determinatedness' (Rothwell *et al.*, 1977).

Convincing period

The transfer of technology from users and intermediaries to manufacturers did however necessitate the introduction of a 'convincing period' of 6–8 months. During this period, the scientific and engineering skills, knowledge and intellectual power of the users and intermediaries which they had built into their innovations had to be transferred. It was found to be difficult to transfer these characteristics especially when equal knowledge, skills, experience and intellectual powers were not present in a manufacturer. One small company, for example, became technically dependent on the user. The 'convincing period' is also the time when the users and intermediaries learn of the expertise of the manufacturer in designing for commercial manufacture and marketing. The period is, therefore, one of incremental learning and trust by both parties enabling them to advance to the next stage of the development. This continuous development created a greater level of commitment by all parties to the achievement of the objective defined by the user. The cooperation between the users, intermediaries and manufacturers expanded the technological base of the manufacturer. In 26 of the innovations there were no entry barriers for the manufacturer to hospital, university and MRC trial facilities and joint testing. Also the combination of clinicians, scientists, engineers and technicians in hospitals working with the manufacturer was evident in the development of 18 of the innovations. Knowledge of these collaborative ventures was diffused throughout the formal and informal networks. This resulted, for instance, in nine users, who had not previously been involved in the development of equipment, identifying the potential manufacturer with whom to work on their innovations. Having developed this expertise and identified the cultural norms expected, continuing interaction through further research programmes or other innovation developments gave the manufacturer a major competitive advantage. In fact, in ten of the innovations in this sample there had been previous cooperation between the manufacturer and the user.

Financing costs

The cooperation also enabled the manufacturer to understand and work within the constraints of the user's capital and revenue budgets. The early identification of the financial parameters within which the user operated helped to ensure the commercial viability of the on-going development was visible. In 27 innovations, this early identification was present. The manufacturers financed the basic and clinically orientated research of the users in nine of the innovations. As well as cash grants, the manufacturers funded research by arranging free use of equipment for research work or loan of equipment. The stimuli for the loan came from two sources. The first was based upon the budget game played by the hospitals, because of the non-transfer of DoH funds from one year to the next. The equipment was loaned until funds could be freed to purchase the equipment or to stop competitors' equipment being purchased. The latter was also achieved by the manufacturer promising to have a more advanced piece of equipment available shortly. The other stimulus was that loan of equipment to teaching hospitals for teaching workshops with international participants creates future sales because clinicians tend to buy, initially at least, the equipment on which they had been trained.

The nature of the management problems associated with this industry funding was illustrated by Dr Parker's unit at University College Hospital's approach to G.D. Searle Ltd in their joint development of the Neo-natal and the Venous Oxygen Monitoring Systems and other developments. The unit realized that, generally, it must typically go through a development period of some 3–5 years to produce a completely new prototype product based on advanced technology. The initial speculative theoretical work alone does not result in industrial funding. The unit, therefore, built into its contract work a surplus for the theoretical work. Because of the time involved in the basic research and, therefore, the cost in terms of man-hours, junior staff tend to be employed in this work. Once the unit has something to show industry, in the form of a clay model or a prototype, it generally attracts funding for further developments. Similarly the scientists can only receive a positive statement from a doctor about the clinical position when something concrete has been developed with which practical experiments can be performed. Because of the clinician's training, and the work environment, it is virtually impossible to speculate about how the body works. Thus the blockages to advances occur at both ends of the innovation process – the invention end and the clinical end. The result of these blockages is that the weight of the funding is in those areas of research which are already well advanced.

An additional problem arises from a bias towards intellectually stimulating and high technology solutions. Market needs that may be solved using low technology and which are beneath the researcher's full potential, tend to be ignored. This bias arises in part from what one's university peers expect and the way in which one's performance is measured, i.e. an intellectually stimulating and challenging paper concerned with an advance in the frontiers of knowledge, rather than a simple solution to a practical problem. This is a major problem for the universities in their relations with industry in that peer evaluation tends to take precedence over the commercial criteria set by industry, especially in terms of the speed of response to commercial stimuli. If the universities are to have a more positive relationship to industry, it seems necessary that performance be measured in the wider context of benefit to the community.

Working capital costs

Some of the cost of prototype development, testing evaluation and marketing were also borne by the user. Examples of these cost transfers were present in all of the case studies examined. In one innovation in particular the supplier, Portex Ltd, incurred part of the development testing and evaluation costs when jointly developing with Graseby Dynamics the diaphragm design for the Respiratory Recording and Monitoring System. Portex, a specialist in the use of plastics for medical use, developed a thin-walled PVC capsule containing PVC foam. The two companies carried out many experiments before settling for a round sensor which was quicker and cheaper to produce on a large scale. Graseby patented the plastic technology and franchised the manufacturer to the plastics specialist. These interactions with users and intermediaries therefore increased the flexibility, quality and cost effectiveness of the manufacturer's resources.

Increasing private returns through market penetration

The increased rate and depth of penetration of the market were developed through:

1 Close collaboration with the user, giving the manufacturer entrée into the international network of researchers. Out of the 11 companies, eight paid retainers to consultants or made them board members to ensure furthering this entrée. Thus a very effective market research facility was created enabling the manufacturer to have some indication of competitive developments, potential new users, uses and the re-innovation required to take advantage of research advances.
2 The medical user acted as a 'reference point' for 27 of the innovations, thus educating potential users in the setting up of clinical trials and the interpretation of results.
3 The user could increase market penetration through the consultant being the signatory to the orders for new equipment and also acting as market and technological gatekeeper outside the centres of excellence.
4 The use made by the manufacturer of the user as the prime communicator was developed to the extent that parts of user's papers or journal articles were quoted in the manufacturer's sales literature, giving the equipment increased credibility and acceptability.

'Inside' and 'outside' product champion

The research concerning the role of the product champion in the innovation process has been principally concerned with the role of the champion *within* the innovating organization. The evidence from the samples studied suggests the need to identify, in addition, the product champions outside the organization. These outside champions, in cooperation with the 'inside product champion', determine the role and the nature of the product development and the final form of the resultant innovation. 'Outside product champions' were coupled with the 'inside product champions' in all of the medical equipment innovations except three. It was found that the status of the majority of these outside product champions, especially where there was more than one outside product champion for an innovation, was matched by the status of the inside product champion. In all the successful innovations, the outside champions, especially where there was more than one for an innovation, were positive driving forces in ensuring that user needs were reflected fully in the final design. The intermediaries (government agencies), acted as major links between the user and the manufacturers.

Conclusion

The relations of the user–designer with the 'intermediaries' and the manufacturers in the medical equipment innovation process, as identified by the research described above, are very creative, economically effective and of significant social benefit. In this sense the process of innovation in medical equipment represents a unique example of the strength of the user–consumer in the development of technology (von Hippel, 1982). It is essential, therefore, that these relations be sustained and developed through creating an organizational climate where they can flourish and an economic setting where the full added value from these interactions can be activated. For this reason the results of the research reported here might suggest the continued encouragement of a highly individualistic contest for the professional prizes of innovation.

References

Allen, T.J. (1977) *Managing the Flow of Technology*. Lancaster: MIT Press.

Blume, S.S. (1965) Towards a theory of biomedical innovation. *Proceedings of the XIVth International Conference on Medical and Biological Engineering and VIIth International Conference in Medical Physics, Espöö, Finland.*

Coleman, J.S., Katz, E. and Menzel, H. (1966) *Diffusion of Innovation*. New York: Free Press.

Crane, D. (1972) *Invisible Colleges: Diffusion of Knowledge in Scientific Communications*. Chicago: The University of Chicago Press.

Freidson, E. (1970) *Professional Dominance: The Social Structure of Medical Care*. Chicago: Aldine.

Gardiner, P. and Rothwell, R. (1985) Tough customers: good designs. *Design Studies*, **6**(1).

Gordon, P.J. (1962) The top management triangle in voluntary hospitals, I and II. *Journal of Academic Management* **4**, 205–14; **5**, 66–75.

Greer, A.L. (1984a) Medical conservation and technological acquisitiveness: The paradox of hospital technology adoptions. In: *The Social Impact of Medical Technology, Vol. 4. Research in the Sociology of Health Care*, (eds) Roth, J.A. and Ruzek, S.B. Greenwich, CT: JAI Press.

Greer, A.L. (1984b) Medical technology and professional dominance theory. *Social Science Medicine*, **18**(10), 809–17.

Harries, J.M. (1981) Development of activities in an action learning set – The role of action learning set advisors. *Training*, **7**(2).

Mansfield, E., Rapoport, J., Romeo, A., Wagner, S. and Beardsley, G. (1977) Social and private returns from industrial innovation. *Quarterly Journal of Economics*, 91.

Myers, L.A. (1983) Information systems in research and development: the technological gatekeeper reconsidered. *R & D Management*, **13**, 4.

Nathan, Robert R. Associates (1978) *Net Rates of Return on Innovations*. Report to the National Science Foundation, October, Vols. 1 and 2. Washington D.C.

Peterson, R.D. and McPhee, C.R. (1973) *Economic Organisation in Medical Equipment and Supply*. Boston, Mass.: Lexington Books.

Reiser, S.J. and Anbar, M. (1984) *The Machine at the Bedside*. Cambridge: Cambridge University Press.

Rogers, E.M. and Shoemaker, F. (1971) *Communication of Innovations*. New York: Free Press.

Rothwell, R., Townsend J., Teubal, M. and Spiller, P. (1977) Some methodological aspects of innovation research. *Omega, The International Journal of Management Science*, **5**(4), 415–24.

Saltman, R.B. and Young, D.W. (1981) The hospital poor equilibrium: an alternative view of the cost containment dilemma. *Journal of Health and Political Policy Law*, **6**, 391–418.

Shaw, B. (1986) The Role of the Interaction between the Manufacturer and the User in the Technological Innovation Process. D.Phil. Thesis, Science Policy Research Unit, University of Sussex.

Tewksbury, J., Crandell, M.S. and Crane, W.E. (1980) Measuring the social benefits of innovation. *Science*, 209.

Tushman, M. and Katz, R. (1980) External communication and project performance: an investigation into the role of gatekeepers. *Management Science*, **26**(11) November.

Von Hippel, E. (1977) The dominant role of the user in semiconductor and electronic sub-assembly process innovation. *IEEE Transactions on Engineering Management*, **EM24**(2), May.

Von Hippel, E. (1982) Appropriability of innovation benefit as a predictor of the source of innovation. *Research Policy*, 11.

9 | Accounting for Patients?: Information Technology and the Implementation of the NHS White Paper

Rod Coombs and David Cooper

Introduction

The NHS is experiencing a radical transformation in its management practices as a result of government intervention and the development of computerized information systems. The overall structure of the various information technology (IT) applications reflects a concern with management of the health service – with resource allocation, efficiency, and budgeting – rather than with clinical applications. Although some systems exist which focus on the clinical information needs of doctors and nurses, they are not receiving the same funding and policy support as management-related systems.

The NHS and Community Care Act (1990) made radical proposals for the use of internal markets to regulate the pattern of health provision and seek greater efficiency. Whilst having distinctive political origins, it is also a further and very obvious manifestation of the managerial direction of development of information systems. Many of the detailed features of the re-organization proposed in the Act – such as trading of clinical services between units, for example – depend crucially on the full-scale implementation of some current pilot schemes to develop management information systems. Prominent amongst these development schemes is the Resource Management Initiative.

Resource management, formerly known as management budgeting, originated from the Griffiths Report on the NHS (1983). Its purpose is to develop procedures which relate information about volumes of work performed by hospital doctors, to information about the costs of that work. The essence of resource management is summed up in a phrase from the Griffiths Report which states that 'the doctors are the natural managers'. The argument is that it is doctors' treatment decisions which result in resources being committed, yet they have no formal responsibility, nor are they accountable (in terms of position in a management hierarchy) for those resources. It is the control of these resources which the NHS Management Board wishes to change. Substantial development projects in resource management have been funded at six national pilot sites but there are also a host of other local initiatives. The White Paper proposed that resource management be 'rolled out' across the rest of the NHS during the period 1984 to 1988.

Our research suggests that there were serious problems in the implementation of resource management. These took the form of technical accounting problems, concerns about the availability of the IT required and confusion about the ownership of resource management. These difficulties with resource management could well lead to the damaging situation whereby accounting logic will frustrate the very goals of the NHS, and the 1989 White Paper *Working for Patients* may indeed become an exercise in 'accounting for patients'. The success of each hospital will be measured by highly dubious performance figures and, despite the apparent concerns of the authors of the White Paper, serious analysis of the quality of patient care will be relegated into the background.

Management in the NHS: the role of accounting

The 1990 Act is attempting to transplant from the private sector to the NHS three alleged rules of management: first, measure and record the inputs to the production process; secondly, measure and record the outputs from the production process; thirdly, make those whose activity most closely determines the ratio of inputs to outputs actually take responsibility for that ratio. The first and second rules translate into budgets and quality-audited workloads. The third rule implies that doctors have also to be managers.

Resource management systems (RMS) attempt to apply the first and second of these rules. They are designed to produce better allocation of resources by relating measures of clinical activity (adjusted to take account of the type of cases being treated) to the costs of that activity. Without such systems, a hospital would find it impossible to produce justifiable charges to other hospitals or health districts for work it has performed. It will also be unable to quote an intelligent price for a treatment requested by a GP or to tender for a service contract from a health authority.

We have examined some of the major developments in resource management at the national pilot sites, and we have been studying in more detail local attempts to develop RMSs in a number of hospitals. These local initiatives follow, but are formally independent of, the national development exercises. Our research has enabled us to identify a series of thorny problems. Some of these are not too surprising to anyone familiar with accounting problems, especially in the NHS context, and indeed they are acknowledged by the people involved. Other problems are more complex and deep rooted, and are less clearly articulated by those involved.

Recognized problems

There have been a series of attempts since the creation of the NHS to make medical practice visible to accountants and manageable through financial logic. Neither the present initiatives nor the past attempts have been able to resolve these problems, many of which are often recognized by the system designers themselves.

The tradition of 'clinical freedom' is central to the professional culture of medicine. This has allowed doctors great autonomy in deciding on treatment regimes, and thus the resources (drugs, surgery, diagnostic tests, nursing staff, bed occupancy, etc.) consumed in treating patients. Although financial constraints have never been absent from the scene, routinely they have been mediated through the everyday practices and culture of professional doctors, rather than through the considered plans of a central hospital or NHS management. There is therefore a conflict between medical traditions and current attempts to institute more bureaucratic and centralized management procedures. In contrast to the traditional, medical mode of control, the idea behind resource management is that the provision of appropriate information to medical staff will regulate their behaviour: if doctors are informed that procedure A costs X and procedure B costs Y then they can more 'rationally' decide which mix of treatments to carry out within an overall budget set at Z.

But how are these costs to be arrived at? Consider the issue of what is to be accounted for. Which doctors 'need' to allocate resources? For example, should all the orthopaedic surgeons in a hospital be treated as a single centre, with one surgeon as the responsible head? This is the approach of at least one of the national sites. Yet at others, each consultant (and their 'firm' of registrars and junior doctors) is treated separately. This system allows comparison between medical practices (the medical audit referred to in the White Paper). But who is to make the comparison? A third approach is to treat each patient or even each treatment as the appropriate focus of attention. Each approach suggests a different pattern of responsibility and decision making and implies a different purpose for the information systems. These issues are unresolved and each creates its own difficulties.

A second problem is how to measure output. Patient care often involves the services of hospitals, GPs, local authorities and the family. If doctors, as a result of the new accounting system, alter their practices, the reduced hospital costs could be more than offset by additional costs due to increased follow-up care by GPs, district nurses, local authority social services or result in lost earnings for family carers. Perhaps medical outcomes or quality of care would be improved by shifts in some treatment patterns, but not in others. Accounting tends to measure the easily measurable and the financial impacts. But such accountings are partial and can lead to resource allocations which all might regard as undesirable.

Another problem is whether doctors should be given information only about variable costs or variable and fixed costs. The former focus attention on performance within a budget period, but the latter can invite them to consider longer term policy issues. When variable costs are a small proportion of total costs, doctors may be encouraged by variable cost information to increase their activity. It is fine in the short term to stimulate more treatments by quoting low prices to GPs and other districts, but there are long-term implications. As congestion increases doctors will point to the need for more facilities. Yet if fixed costs were included in an average cost figure for a treatment, doctors would quickly see through the arbitrary nature of such allocations and the cost information would be discredited.

Finally, how is a distinction to be made between controllable and non-controllable costs? Drugs are relatively controllable and attract a lot of attention but are frequently a small proportion of total costs. Ward-related costs, like nursing manpower, are much greater, but current management structures give doctors little control over them. Should doctors be responsible for items they cannot control. And if they are not given responsibility, who should be?

Unacknowledged problems

IT. Whilst the problems listed above might perhaps be regarded as 'soluble' within the intellectual framework of accounting, and are seen in this light by many of the professional managers involved, there are two other problems which have a more complex character. The first of these concerns the development of the information technology systems. To the extent it is recognized, IT is seen as a technical and financial problem. The second issue is seen by the participants but is regarded as a political problem. It concerns the real and perceived relationships of control between doctors and managers. In fact, we would also argue that the technical and the political dimensions of the two problems are more intricately connected than this. Let us first, however, examine them separately.

The IT problem is one of introducing activity-measuring and cost-allocating systems into all hospital departments. The systems then feed back all the information collected into a 'black box' piece of software which adds up the component costs and links them to particular types of illness or treatment, and particular patients and doctors. The various national sites have developed systems with different hardware, using different software and being advised by different consultants. It is intended that each system will be compatible with a general commitment to case mix accounting. Yet it is already clear that the hardware suppliers and the software consultancy companies will be competing with systems with quite different specifications.

The original national sites have had considerable resources, provided both by the NHS Management Board and the firms keen to obtain access to an expanding market. Our observations at the local sites suggest that the resource requirements are consistently underestimated, even when the local management only wish to modify an existing system. Developing and installing these systems, especially if the output is to be widely available to doctors in a user-friendly form, costs a great deal – enough to make the IT suppliers treat the NHS as a serious growth market for the rest of the century. But will the hospitals have the necessary money?

Hospitals are operating in conditions where the government wishes to limit total NHS expenditure. In addition, hospital management are concerned to avoid accusations of sacrificing patient care and the expansion of treatment programmes for investment in 'bureaucracy' and their own empires. In the context of a history of cash limits, most computer systems are regarded as being orientated to control and cost savings. There is little belief amongst clinicians in the view that RMS can augment the quality of medical diagnosis and patient care. In such a situation, there are few champions for the investment in IT required for resource management.

Ownership of RMSs. The second unrecognized problem concerns 'ownership' of the RMS. Here there is a diversity of opinion and practice in the hospitals we have studied. At one extreme, and most consistent with the stated philosophy of the White Paper, is 'doctor ownership'. This official version of resource management 'sells' the package to doctors by building into the software significant amounts of patient information which are clinically useful to the doctor in carrying out his professional responsibilities. Indeed in our research we observed the embryos of some potentially very exciting ways in which IT-based medical information, provided through a RMS, could give doctors the ability to carry out detailed epidemiological research, in the context of formal Medical Audit. Such developments could genuinely increase the capability of medical research and thus the quality of patient care.

The doctor-ownership model of resource management has a 'political' dimension in that it aims to overcome doctors' resistance by allowing them to participate in the design of the systems. The next step is to put the information in appealing formats on a PC on the doctor's desk. This approach is predicated on the hope that, once hooked, doctors will naturally progress to viewing the financial and management issues raised by the systems as interesting and pertinent problems for them to address. The long-term logic of this model is that of the doctor-as-manager.

Finance department ownership. At the other extreme, and more consistent with what we have observed in the local initiatives, is an approach which involves 'finance department ownership'. In this model the information systems are designed by 'experts' and are based on more conventional accounting concepts. They tend to play down clinical information. They are relatively cheap with an emphasis on accounting control information designed for professional accountants. The RMS becomes a budgetary control system for the hospital. Cost control is the focus. This also implies that clinical policy is more directly driven by Unit General Managers who use the information to set the agenda for clinical debates. Clinicians are invited to be involved once the system is operating.

This latter approach is at odds with some important features of the Act's stated philosophy, but has a strong inertial force behind it which derives from accounting orthodoxy, medical indifference to the more radical system, and, finally, lower cost. This is where the financial and ownership dimensions of the IT 'strategy' can contradict each other. The finance department ownership approach is the default option. It is very likely to occur if resource management is implemented without adequate resources and local clinician commitment.

Risks and uncertainties

We are not arguing here for or against the 1990 Act's proposals. What we are pointing out is that there are important features of the situation into which they are being deployed and which may well result in the worst of all worlds. If there is a loss of nerve in the IT investment programme, and if the mutual suspicions of accountants and doctors prevail, systems could result which tighten financial control without sufficient doctor involvement to adequately confront issues of the quality of medical outcomes and the patterns of care between patient groups. There would be a wholly spurious and even damaging increase in financial rectitude in the NHS.

The final complicating twist in the story is that the technical and the political aspects of the problem are not separate at all but are actually being increasingly tied together. In any hospital that attempts to develop or install a RMS there is an immediate problem of designing the software, the report formats and the distribution of the hardware. The design has a built-in concept of management structures and responsibilities. Thus the attitudes to the political issue of medical and managerial responsibilities and their location come under the spotlight straight away.

A key factor therefore in the future evolution of resource management is the uncertainty within the medical profession as to how far it is willing to move in adjusting its values and culture in a direction which accommodates 'managerial' aspects. This factor will certainly have a profound influence on whether the doctor-ownership model or the finance department-ownership model becomes dominant. The White Paper's emphasis on internal markets and trading of clinical services between districts has brought this issue sharply into focus. Groups of doctors are now being confronted with the threats and the opportunities associated with a future environment in which competitiveness will be an increasingly common yardstick for the evaluation of providers of medical services. This will be true for individual doctors, for groups of doctors in the same specialty, for hospitals, and for District Health Authorities. These competitive relations are intertwined with the changes in control procedures which the IT systems will usher in.

It has been argued elsewhere (Coombs, 1987), in the context of the Swedish health system, that there is some reason to expect the medical profession to at least consider the possibility of responding to this challenge by annexing management and incorporating it into a revised definition of medical practice, thus overturning some of the shibboleths of 'clinical freedom'. But the recent actions of some doctors in the NHS indicate the presence of contradictory views. For example, doctors in the six pilot sites for resource management have declared themselves to be opposed to their hospitals 'opting out' into self-management under the terms of the Act, but have at the same time endorsed their commitment to the resource management experiments.

Conclusion

Our analysis of developments in the application of IT to management information systems in the NHS (for more details, see Bloomfield and Coombs, 1989), has illustrated the dynamics of change as central authorities intervene to increase visibility and control and to incite competitiveness as an organizing force in the relationships between sub-units of the NHS. This attempted intervention utilizes a variety of weapons ranging from direct political debate in the public domain, through administrative force majeure in the re-organization of contracts etc., and, most importantly for our analysis, the systematic strengthening of the IT-based information systems which are used by personnel at all levels in the NHS to 'manage' their own and others' activities. Resource management has been our example of this.

This attempt to reshape control and competition in the NHS plainly involves an instrumental stance toward the culture of the NHS. There is a desire to change the way doctors in particular 'see' the NHS and the way they think about its goals and their own work. What is less plain, equally powerful, and therefore very relevant to organizations which are not as publicly visible as the NHS, is the way the shift in practice is being attempted through the creation of specific information systems which privilege particular kinds of information and reinforce certain forms of knowledge about what the NHS is and what its goals and procedures should be. A new common sense for people involved in medical work is being negotiated through the apparently arcane technical discussions of software packages and accounting conventions and a significant change in organizational culture seems to be the intention.

It will be clear from what we have said, however, that this instrumental attitude to the culture of the NHS is unlikely to produce unambiguous consequences. There are divergent but strongly held views within the NHS about its goals and its modes of operation. These views are deeply embedded in the cultures of professional groups within the NHS. Thus the outcome of the intervention will depart from the intentions of the interveners in some respects, and be reshaped through the multiple cultures of the various groups in the NHS who are the targets of the intervention. The NHS is about to learn a fourth rule of management; arguments about information systems are arguments about the very goals of the organization. High performing organizations tend to have a fit between their goals, their management structures and their information systems. It is time to connect these to the goals of the NHS and the question of whether health care is a consumer good or a citizen's right. Behind the technical arguments lie fundamental social policy and political issues. IT systems will not – and should not – provide a 'fix' for these problems.

References

Bloomfield, B. and Coombs, R. (1989) Information Technology, Control and Power: The Centralisation and De-Centralisation Debate Re-visited. 'CROMTEC Working Paper'. Manchester: School of Management, UMIST.

Coombs, R. (1987) Accounting for the control of doctors: management information systems in Swedish hospitals. *Accounting, Organisations and Society*, **12**(4), 389–404.

Department of Health (1989) *Working for Patients*. London: HMSO.

Griffiths, R. (1983) *Report of the NHS Management Inquiry*. London: DHSS.

10 | Modes of Innovation in Management Information Systems

Michael Dent, Ruth Green, Judy Smith and David Cox

Introduction

This chapter describes and analyses the implementation of computer-based management information systems within four health districts. It is set against the background of a major reorganization of the system of health service management. In turn this change was intended to generate a new demand for the information as a consequence of the Government's acceptance and immediate implementation of the Griffiths Management Inquiry. The key point of the Griffiths Report was its recommendation that the management structure of the NHS should be in future based on a system of general management rather than the previous model of 'consensus management'.

General management was intended to ensure that specified managers were responsible (accountable) for the coordination and control of the health service at all levels and that the management structure was integrated into a single line of command from the hospital and community units through to the district general manager. At each level someone was to be responsible for setting objectives and ensuring they were attained. The system of general management was also implemented within the offices of the Regional Health Authorities (RHAs) and the whole system of health service management was the global responsibility of NHS Supervisory and Management Boards at the national level. Here, however, we are concerned only with the situation within the districts.

With the implementation of the new system of general management came the imperative for districts to have greater control over their resources and the greater need for accurate, up-to-date information; without these the concept of general management would seem meaningless, for they are the means by which decisions are made. Under these new management arrangements the key measures of performance related to financial resources, manpower and patient activity; these had always been concerns of the NHS but not in the integral way they now became. This assertion can be substantiated by reference to the 1981 Commons Select Committee on Social Services which criticized the then DHSS for not being clear about its health service aims when deciding to increase or decrease expenditure, and in lacking the means of accurately monitoring the outcomes of any such decisions. In that same year the Commons Public Accounts Committee were also critical of the ineffectiveness of the NHS systems of monitoring and controlling staffing (i.e. manpower).[1]

This concern of Parliament with management information leads us again to the central focus of this chapter, computer-based management information systems. The region in which the research reported here took place was committed to implementing a set of corporate computer systems designed to provide comprehensive informational support to the district general managers as well as to the regional authorities and the NHS Management and Supervisory Boards by April 1987. This chapter draws upon case study observation of this process in four health authorities carried out in the late summer of 1986. The research was concerned to find out how the district managements had prepared for, and were responding to, the implementation of three corporate computer systems with particular reference to a manpower information system. We were concerned to analyse the implementation processes in terms of the strategies of the management groups involved. For this reason we start with a discussion of the concept of management strategies before moving on to describe in more detail the organizational context of the study and the three corporate computer systems with which we were concerned. The main part of the chapter, however, concentrates on describing and analysing the processes and procedures adopted within each of the four districts in order to try to implement these management information systems within the intended time-scale. The chapter ends with a summary of our argument and conclusions.

Management strategies

Our main theoretical interest related to the management strategies adopted by district managers in relation to the implementation of the corporate computer systems. Following Child (1985a), managerial strategies can be seen as the conceptual linkage between structure, action and outcome as played out within the arena of the work organization. This is not to assert, however, that management strategies *determine* outcomes, rather that they constitute a *mediation* between the imperatives of 'capitalism', the corporate intentions of the organization and the labour process outcomes (Child,

1985a, p. 113). There is no implication that the strategies in practice will always be coherent, nor that the implementation of the policies will reflect precisely the intentions of management (which are rarely unitary in any organization). In Child's model there is the assumption that the strategies will have a dominant effect on organizational outcomes in the private sector. However he does not envisage this as always being the case in the non-market public sector where management has never had the apparent autonomy and power possessed by their counterparts in industry. In the NHS this is largely because of the influence of the professions in health service decision making.

Contrarily we would argue that the concept of management strategy does have an explanatory role to play in the analysis of organizational outcomes within the public sector, although unlike 'enterprises funded by private capital' (Child, 1985a, p. 108) these strategies are more policy- than market-driven. We were also concerned with utilizing the concept of *management strategy* as a means of developing a comparative schema between the four health districts studied within the health service.

The organizational context of the study

It is important to present details of the organizational context of the health districts at the time of the planned implementation of the computer systems, for management strategies within the health service are not premised on fundamental capitalistic objectives (Child, 1985a, p. 112), or at least not directly so, but on policy considerations.

In 1980, long before the setting up of the Griffiths Inquiry, a joint NHS/DHSS Steering Group on Health Services Information had been set up to examine and make recommendations regarding management information requirements within the health service. The steering group was chaired by Mrs Edith Körner, whose name became indelibly linked with the new system of management information collection to be discussed later. The work of the 'Group' had two main thrusts:

(1) to carry out a comprehensive review of the data content of NHS information systems; and
(2) the development of an environment which encouraged the efficient collection, processing and analysis of data and the effective transmission and use of information. (Mason, 1984, p. 24).

The work of the steering group was divided between eight working groups covering most aspects of the work of the health service supported by a range of research and development projects. The recommendations contained within the subsequent reports became a mandatory requirement in April 1984. The deadline for the implementation of some recommendations was April 1987 and for others, April 1988 (*British Journal of*

Healthcare Computing, Summer, 1984, p. 5). Meeting these deadlines by any means (manual or automated) became an important political requirement fed down from Ministers to regional chair(wo)men and regional general managers.

The new requirements for gathering and storing health service data resulting from the implementation of the Körner recommendations could only be met adequately with computer support (Windsor, 1984, p. 3). The responses of the districts studied here to these two demands was largely determined by policy made by senior regional management: districts rarely implemented computer systems independently of the Regional Health Authorities (excepting the purchase of micros) for the latter held all the computer-related resources. In the region with which we were concerned, the senior management adopted the policy of developing and implementing a set of corporate computer systems designed to capture and process all the data required to meet the specific recommendations set out in the Körner Reports. Moreover, these systems were designed to provide an integrated district management information system, at least eventually.

The corporate systems strategy was largely the consequence of the high level of resource commitment given to the development of hospital and health service computer systems by this region throughout the 1970s as part of the NHS Experimental Computer Programme which ended in 1981 (Dent, 1988). The implementation of corporate systems throughout the region resulted from the application of the logic of fully exploiting the expensive computer facilities and technical staff that had already been developed rather than any prima facie rationale that corporate *computer* systems were strictly necessary to support corporate *information* systems. In consequence, there was room for the districts to be unconvinced of the region's corporate computer strategy and to favour instead implementing other computer systems. The region avoided this possibility by 'top-slicing' the districts' budgets by the amount required for the corporate systems implementation programme and offering the districts a 100% discount on the basic systems.

Paradoxically, the development and implementation of these corporate systems was constrained by the Government's imposition of the April 1987 deadline for the introduction of the Körner recommendations. This meant that nationally the regions had to get the computer systems implemented very rapidly in order to meet the Körner requirements. In consequence, all the other facets of the corporate systems and their role in supporting district management information systems had to be left in various degrees of abeyance. This situation gave rise to great uncertainty and the introduction of the corporate computer systems became a contested issue between the different levels of management within and between region and districts.

Before discussing the nature of these inter-managerial relations we first need to say rather more about the three corporate computer systems with which we are concerned.

The corporate computer systems

The three corporate computer systems covered broadly accounting, patient administration and manpower. For our purposes we have called them (fictitiously) the

(i)   Resource Management System (RMS);
(ii) Patient Administration and Information System (PAIS); and the
(iii) Manpower Information System (MPIS).

All three systems were essentially database systems which operationally captured data with the intention of providing information for local and national management and administrative purposes. Together the systems covered manpower, finance and (patient) activity. We shall now briefly describe each system in turn.

RMS. RMS was essentially a realtime 'update' of an existing system. It was a financial information system with a core accounting module designed to provide the basic costing data for management reports, including manpower and patient activity. The system was intended, at least initially, to run on the RHA's ICL mainframe machine on a bureau basis. At the time of the research, the RMS system was being piloted at a small number of health districts and was due to be implemented throughout the region in 1986. It was decided at a late stage, however, by senior regional officers to postpone the implementation until the system had been piloted for a further period of time in order to eradicate certain design faults. This effectively delayed the implementation process another year and beyond the 'Körner' deadline. Despite this setback the central importance of financial information and control for the management of the health service ensured the system a core position in the matrix of the region's corporate computer systems.

PAIS. PAIS was the system that had been most developed and evaluated within the health service. The system consisted of three modules:

● an index of all patients (past and present)
● details of in-patient-related activity
● details of out-patient-related activity

The system was a wholly *operational* one, and was unable to provide much in the way of aggregate data necessary for management planning. A fourth 'Patient Information System' module was in the process of being introduced. The system ran on ICL mainframe equipment located within the districts.

MPIS. Unlike the other two systems MPIS was a wholly new initiative and did not derive directly from systems developed during the NHS Experimental Computer Programme. The system was the 'brain-child' of a member of the region's computer staff and was initiated by the region within the South district (one of the districts included in the research – see below) in the early 1980s. The need for the system was generally recognized by the regional officers concerned with computing policy, because the pre-existing manpower system was (a) not a realtime system nor (b) was it able to provide all the information required by the DHSS and Region following the implementation of the Körner recommendations (cf. Third Report, 1984, especially Recommendations 22–25, p. 32). Moreover, it was the view of the region's computer services division that they had to find some means of providing districts with an 'in-house' manpower system if they were to remain in control of future computer developments and not be superseded by districts buying their own systems from other sources.

MPIS was ultimately intended to consist of five phases, or modules:

I   An index of all staff to replace the previous non-interactive system.
II Staff qualifications and training.
III Details of posts (this module was to provide the information required for the Körner Reports and some additional information for the DHSS).
IV A budgeting module, relating manpower requirements to resources and workloads.
V   An integrated personnel and pay-roll system, including facilities for maintaining records of sickness and absences.

At the time of the research these phases were being developed out of sequence because of the priority of fulfilling the requirements of the Körner recommendations. As with RMS systems the system was run as a bureau service based on the region's ICL mainframe.

The three corporate systems were piloted and implemented independently of one another. In the case of PAIS this was of little consequence, but this was not the case with the MPIS and RMS systems; these systems had been intended to be integrated in order that the financial consequences of manpower planning and control could be fully calculable.

Research design and methodology

We now turn to the four health districts that constituted our case studies. These districts were selected according to (a) size and complexity and (b) stage of implementation of the MPIS system, including an example of an early, middle-ranking and late adopter of the system. The criteria for selection are discussed in more detail in the next section. In order to maintain the anonymity of the four districts included in the study they have been renamed by the cardinal points of the compass, North, South, East and West.

The research was carried out over four months (June–September) in 1986. The methods of investigation used were those of:

- tape recorded semi-structured interviews with key members of management and staff involved with the implementation and use of the corporate computer systems and with district computer development generally
- unstructured interviews with members of the regional corporate computer systems implementation team
- observations of district meetings (steering and advisory groups)
- an analysis of regional and district documents and minutes of meetings related to the corporate computer systems and their implementation
- presentation of the research findings to the individual districts in order to allow for criticism and comments

The methodology was qualitive in design with each technique being used to inform and corroborate the data collected by the others in a way similar to 'triangulation' (Pettigrew, 1979).

The four districts

The size of the districts and the complexity of their organizational structures were employed as the basic criteria for selection and comparison of the four case studies. In addition, the stage of MPIS implementation was also taken into consideration. The criteria were adopted on the grounds of operational simplicity and warranted on the grounds that size and complexity have generally been found to be of strategic importance in the analysis and development of management control systems (e.g. Child, 1973, pp. 237–9; 1985b, pp. 59–61), while selection according to stage of implementation meant we were able to gain an understanding of the interplay between management reorganization and systems implementation on a comparative basis. In this section we will discuss the structural dimensions of the four districts, while the comparative dimension will be dealt with later.

Size was measured in terms of the number of the home population within the community the district served plus the number of staff employed within the authority (Appendix 10.1). Complexity was interpreted to mean the number of management and hospital/community units (Appendix 10.2). The four districts can be usefully characterized for comparative purposes as in Table 10.1.

West and South Districts were the two largest districts. Moreover, West had the simplest structure of all the districts studied (two unit general managers (UGM) with four hospital/community units). The most complex district was South East (a three-UGM structure with six hospital/community units).

Table 10.1 Characteristics of the four districts

Complexity	Size of district	
	Small	Large
Simple	North	West
Complex	East	South

Note: Small/large and Simple/complex are used here as relative and not absolute terms.

Management structure, strategies and the corporate systems

We found from interviews that the corporate systems were only attractive to district managers in so far as the systems were perceived as being able to deliver an improved local service. This was widely believed to be the case with PAIS. The RMS system was recognized by the finance people as promising to be an improvement on the current batch standard accounting system. This was not the case with the manpower system (MPIS). While it was designed *ultimately* to offer a comprehensive and timely realtime service, the short-term priority of the regional systems' personnel was to develop and implement only those modules necessary for the Körner and DHSS Reports. In consequence, the MPIS system was generally viewed by the managers as having little relevance for their local purposes, at least for the present.

This generalization, however, oversimplifies matters and the four districts presented considerable variation in their managements' policies and responses to the implementation of the corporate computer systems. The positions in each of the districts studied will be explored in turn in order to identify and analyse the nature of these variations.

South District. This district was well advanced in its implementation of the 'Griffiths' management structures; only the North District was more advanced. Under these new arrangements the management of the district was coordinated through the General Managers Group (consisting of the DGM and three UGMs), while the old district management team (DMT) had been reconstituted as the Chief Officers Group (COG) and had advisory powers only. The information strategy of the district was the broad responsibility of the District Treasurer.

Up until mid-1986 implementing the MPIS system had been wholly delegated to the District Nursing Officer and treated, in effect, as a separate development independent of other computer-based information systems within the district. This 'separate development' approach was not so different from that adopted by the other three districts *except* that elsewhere MPIS was delegated to district personnel officers rather than nursing officers, i.e. delegated *within* the administrative hierarchy rather than *across* to the professional domain of nursing management with the resulting attenuation of organizational control. This arrangement we refer to as 'systems isolationism' and it resulted from certain historical factors peculiar to that district.

The modules of the MPIS system were piloted at this district and the system had been implemented, at least partially, at the unit as well as district level. Yet despite this level of development, the system was not much used within the district. Part of the reason for this was the inadequate state of relations between the manpower office and the finance department. MPIS was intended to use a coding system in common with the district's finance (manual) system, but the finance people involved were unwilling to give the time necessary to ensure the system's coding was accurate and up-to-date. In consequence the MPIS outputs were not always as accurate as they would otherwise have been.

A more fundamental reason for the system's isolation, however, was the district personnel officer's rejection of the system early in its development on the grounds that the development and implementation of the system was too slow. Thus, for most of the system's history within this district, the unusual situation existed where the personnel department was not responsible for manpower information. Instead, and as already stated, the system became the responsibility of the District Nursing Officer (DNO). The work associated with the operation of the system was carried out within a small manpower office where the district computer terminals were located. The main rationale for this arrangement (given the personnel officer's rejection of the system) related to the fact that the DNO had had experience of implementing two nursing manpower systems previously.

The DNO had, in addition to establishing the manpower office, set up a small cadre of liaison officers comprising of both nursing managers and administrators (one of each per unit). These persons had the responsibility of coordinating the implementation of the system within the unit for which they were responsible. However, as already indicated, the system lacked any effective management support, being largely (but not totally) ignored by both district and unit management. This situation only began to change when the Körner deadline was less than 12 months away. Only then was there any attempt made to prioritize the implementation and utilization of the system. This renewed interest in the system coincided with the early retirement of the DNO and his replacement by a newly appointed district information officer (subordinate to the district treasurer). The information officer was intended to fully implement the MPIS system. To achieve this, the officer planned to bring the system back into the management structure and initially he tried to get the district personnel officer to re-adopt the system, but when this failed one of the unit personnel officers was persuaded to take on the responsibility.

North District. This district was the most advanced in its programme of reorganization following the Griffiths and Körner Reports. It had implemented the Griffiths management arrangements down to unit management level by mid-1986 and had appointed an information officer (coordinator) by the same time. Unlike the South District (above) there was already a computer adviser in post. The general management arrangements were coordinated via a fortnightly general managers' meeting which included, in addition to the DGM and UGMs, the Treasurer and the Director of Planning and Information. The old DMT survived primarily as the means of consultation with the health professionals. Information strategy had a high priority and was the major item on the agenda of every third general managers' meeting (approximately at six-weekly intervals) when the information officer joined the group in an advisory capacity.

The DGM had adopted a strong corporate approach (which we came to refer to as 'district corporacy'). It was his view that the organizational objective of delivering health care efficiently and effectively was best achieved when there was a recognition of the mutuality of interests between the constituent parts of the service where otherwise this would not necessarily be the case with UGMs and others at unit level bidding against each other for limited resources (e.g. acute and community). In order to facilitate a common commitment to this corporacy the DGM had implemented the policy of devolving a considerable amount of decision making down to the units and strongly encouraged the UGMs and other officers to take an active role in the development of information and computing strategies. This corporate policy gave rise to a high degree of commitment from the senior management to the development of information technology and ensured the MPIS system was viewed fairly positively. Moreover, the treasurer's department were involved with the implementation of the system right from the beginning, so that the problems of compatibility as between MPIS and RMS, a serious problem at the South District, was minimized.

The corporatist strategy, however, was not without its problems. In part this was because resource constraints made it impossible for the district to provide the computer equipment to the unit managers and their staff necessary in order to set up an integrated computer-based information system.

In addition, it was also the case that one occupational group – the nurses – had serious reservations regarding the management re-organization in general and the requirements of the Körner recommendations in particular. Whether this meant the nurses were antipathetic to the MPIS system or not was unclear for they were unrepresented on the systems steering group and on the district committees dealing with information strategy. It was, however, reported by different members of these committees that it was likely to prove difficult to gain the cooperation of the nursing staff as they were reported to be exhibiting a general lack of enthusiasm for gathering new and possibly complicated data for the MPIS system. This failure to involve the nursing staff was a major shortcoming, for the nurses are the largest occupational grouping within the NHS and their absence from the system seriously undermined its usefulness.

East District. This district adopted a relatively slow and measured response to the demands for management change. The 'Griffiths' arrangements were being implemented in a minimalist way as they were based on the pre-existing Units (Appendix 10.2) that were being reorganized. In connection with the development of the district's information strategy very little consideration had at that time been given to the subject. The authority had only recently appointed an information officer to overview this and related developments.

In relation to the implementation of the MPIS system the response of the East District was a 'low key' but not an antipathetic one. We characterized it as one of 'committed pragmatism'. The district's approach was to follow the Region's policy regarding the adoption and implementation of the system but without any great enthusiasm for it. It would be wrong, however, to interpret this as apathy. The general attitude among those involved was one of 'get the system implemented first, explore its uses later'.

The MPIS system was implemented quickly and effectively under the leadership of the deputy district personnel officer. As in the North District, the implementation process directly involved unit staff from an early stage. This participation was further extended with the staff within the units being directly involved in the practical preparations for the adoption of the system. This involvement included – in contrast to the North District – the nursing staff. This was the consequence of the limited numbers of people available for this work but it did result in a high degree of cooperation and commitment from the staff involved.

It was possible, of course, that the generally agnostic attitude of managers and personnel officers to the MPIS system would change once the 'Griffiths' restructuring was completed and all the general management posts had been filled. Then there would be a distinct possibility of an increase in demand for manpower information. At the time of the research, however, this was not the case. The MPIS represented part of the management information systems (MIS) infrastructure deemed necessary by the Region for the new era following the implementation of the Griffiths and Körner Reports. Under these circumstances the 'committed pragmatic' approach proved to be an effective strategy; it not only ensured that virtually all the necessary arrangements for the implementation of the system were completed within the Körner timescale but it was the means by which the personnel officers were able to effectively motivate and train staff.

West District. This district was one of the larger ones and according to the figures available to us employed substantially more staff than any of the other districts included in our study (see Appendix 10.1). Like the smaller East District it too had yet to complete the reorganization of its management structures. Part of the reason for this situation was that the district management were taking the opportunity of the reorganization to simplify the internal management structures by reducing the pre-existing four site-base units of management to a two-unit structure – 'acute' and 'community & longstay' (see Appendix 10.2).

There had been a pre-existing computer committee that had advised the DMT on computing matters. But this was to be superseded by a more information-orientated committee better able to respond to the demands of the Körner Reports in which the emphasis was on the data and information required for effective health service management rather than on what computer equipment constituted the 'best buy' for the district. This had been the main diet of the original computer committee. Within the new climate the district management were beginning to take a lead in establishing broad policy regarding healthcare information. As part of this policy a specific district-wide coordinating body was set up in September 1986, known as the Körner Committee.

The implementation of the corporate computer systems which were intended to support the new Körner-style information systems were, however, each treated as wholly separate activities with little in common with each other, least of all membership. In connection with the MPIS system, we came to refer to this arrangement as 'pragmatic separatism'; it had certain similarities with those of the East District (the pragmatism) while also demonstrating some characteristics more like those found in the South district, i.e. a lack of integration.

MPIS was treated as a separate development within the district and implementation was placed under the control of the district personnel officer. The steering group was relatively small and the members were selected for their expertise rather than their ability to represent constituencies (e.g. units). This strategy ensured that the implementation programme was completed on schedule, but this was achieved with little consultation with members of the district and unit management. The result was that it was unclear whether the arrangements would in practice be acceptable to other managers within the district.

Review

In this brief review of the four districts we have identified the basic management strategies employed. These strategies were developed largely, but not wholly, in response to the circumstances the districts found themselves in at the time the system was being implemented. The chief considerations here were as follows:

- The extent to which the general management arrangements had been implemented and the new posts filled.

Table 10.2 Size and MPIS implementation

Stage of implementation	Size of district	
	Larger	Smaller
Advanced	South District	North District
Intermediate and late	West District (late)	East District (intermediate)

- The requirement to develop an information strategy that would specifically ensure that the information required by the Körner recommendations would be systematically collected.
- Whether the districts had plans to develop appropriate management information systems to underpin the new general management arrangements.

The corporate systems themselves were designed to support these developments but because the systems were being introduced prior to the districts completing their own organizational rearrangements the integration of the 'parts' of the general management strategy was problematic. Rather than assisting in the process of reorganization the programme of computer implementation was an additional burden, giving rise to *ad hoc* solutions rather than systematic arrangements integrated within a broader information management strategy.

District comparisons

Differences between the districts' management strategies, implementation arrangements and the levels of acceptability of the MPIS corporate system related directly, as we have already indicated, to the degree to which the districts had implemented the new general management arrangements. In addition, however, the structural variable of size was found to be important in influencing the likelihood of an effective implementation of the MPIS system (see Table 10.2). Complexity, by contrast, was an ambiguous indicator largely because of the timings of the studies, i.e. when the numbers and organization of the management units were in the process of being changed as part of the new Griffiths arrangements (1983). In this section we present a comparative analysis of the districts in order to develop the analysis of the inter-relationship between strategies and organizational structure further.

South and North Districts

There were some similarities between these two districts in as much as they had both largely implemented the Griffiths management arrangements and had appointed information officers. The General Managers

Group in both Districts was similar and there was a prima facie similarity between the Chief Officers Group (COG) of the South District and the reincarnated 'DMT' at the North District. There were nevertheless fundamental differences in management arrangements and cultures between the two districts. Firstly, the North District was relatively new, having come into existence in the wake of the demise of the Area Health Authorities (AHAs) in 1982. This was not the case with the South District which, like most districts, was established as part of the 1974 reorganization of the NHS (Ham, 1985, p. 26). In consequence, the DGM at the North District was able to use the Griffiths reorganization as an opportunity to implement his own programme of District corporacy (see p. 135 above) for, unlike his opposite number at the South District, he was not confronted with a large district with a well-established management structure with its associated cliques and cabals (Burns, 1955). As part of his general strategy, the DGM at the North District was committed to the development of integrated information systems to under-pin his corporate model. It was in consequence of this 'district corporacy' that the implementation of the corporate computer systems, including the MPIS, were that much easier than at the South District where the circumstances and the strategies were very different.

The South District management lacked any tangible corporate ethos. The district was larger (see Appendix 10.1) and mainly served an inner city area which, given the social and economic problems associated with such areas, further compounded its difficulties. Moreover, the district did not have the opportunity of starting with a 'clean slate' as had been the case with the newly established North District, but had to accommodate to the reorganization and computerization of a well-established management team. Against this background the introduction of the corporate computer systems tended to be seen by these managers as a luxury they could well afford to do without unless the systems produced immediate operationally beneficial results. In the case of both the PAIS and RMS systems the general belief of management was that these might well meet this criterion of usefulness. The MPIS system, by contrast, was generally viewed as being of very limited or no use. As explained earlier (p. 134) this was related as much to the *isolationism* of the system within the district as to any technical shortcomings the system suffered. It was rejected by the personnel officer, ignored by most managers and only implemented at all because it had been delegated, by the DGM, to the district nursing officer who could operate largely independently of the administrative hierarchy. To have piloted such a system in this district, as the regional computer services did, can only be rationalized on the old adage that 'if it will work there, it will work anywhere'. The implementation of the system was not successful simply because the district and unit management and staff outside the cadre of the MPIS steering group members were unable or unwilling to give the necessary priority to the implementation programme.

In summary, the South District was very limited in its ability to develop (pilot) the MPIS system for largely historical and contextual factors. The North District, by contrast, was able to innovate with little (or less) danger of serious organizational problems, being of a relatively small size and in possession of an integrated management structure and ideology.

East and West Districts

East and West Districts, while not being at dissimilar stages of MPIS implementation, exhibited very different approaches towards the implementation of the system. In large part, the explanation for the differences was related to the differences in organizational size; the role of management culture, whilst contributing to the variation between the two districts, was less of a causal factor than had been the case with the North and South Districts.

East District was the smaller district of the two. At the time of the research it was in the process of implementing the Griffiths management reorganization. This, however, did not involve any major changes to the pre-existing unit arrangements. An information officer had recently been appointed but had not yet taken any direct role in the implementation of MPIS within the district. Nor was there any attempt made by the senior management to incorporate systems into any district strategy. Instead the managerial strategy was wholly a pragmatic one of implementing the system and postponing consideration of what use it might be until a later date. In adopting this strategy the district and, more specifically, the personnel department, had successfully implemented the first (and then only available) phase of MPIS.

The West District was at a similar stage in implementing the Griffiths arrangements but here there was rather more uncertainty as to the consequences. The unit structure was to be revised from a four-unit to a simpler two-unit structure (see Appendix 10.2). An information officer had been appointed but, similarly to the East District, had not yet become sufficiently involved with MPIS to influence matters. The implementation programme was directly the responsibility of the personnel department, as was the case of the East District. But unlike that district, the MPIS Steering Group contained only district personnel, i.e. it excluded unit staff. Consideration of how best the system might be used in the district or what role the system might play in the district's information strategy was for the time being postponed. The minimal involvement or consultation with others was seen as the best way of achieving the speediest implementation of the system.

The result was a success in principle, without the participants having any real knowledge as to whether the arrangements for the system's implementation would work in practice. This situation came about because in the period leading up to the implementation of the new management arrangements (Griffiths) there were no persons outside the MPIS

Steering Group with any specific interest in manpower information systems. Moreover, being a large district, the opportunities for pragmatism of the kind identified at East District were limited. Each manager/officer was too constrained by the priorities pertaining to their discipline/function to be able to contribute effectively to the implementation of MPIS. Relatedly, the priority of higher management was at that time with the implementation of the Körner recommendations and until that was achieved the demands of any individual computer-based system, or their integration, were seen as taking a lower priority.

Both East and West Districts had organized for the implementation of the MPIS system but solely on pragmatic grounds. The system was part of the region's package of corporate systems and for that reason, rather than any intrinsic qualities of the system itself, the districts made arrangements for its implementation. In the case of the East District, the personnel department made a virtue out of limited resources by involving as many people as possible in the preparations for the system's implementation and thereby ensuring maximum participation and consultation. By contrast, the personnel department in the West District was far more isolationist in its approach and the implementation process was very much carried out from above; being a larger district, the West was denied the flexibility open to the East District due to the problems associated with the coordination between units and departments. These were problems which were being further exacerbated by the district reorganization being carried out at that time.

The Four Districts: Summary

Computers can play a role as the technology that enables districts to avoid the bureaucratization tendency inherent in large-scale organizations. Computer-based management information systems as rapid communicators and analysers of information can simplify the problems of coordination and control confronting management within large complex organizations. To achieve this state of affairs, however, the system has first to be implemented. The systems' implementors within the larger districts were confronted with greater problems than their colleagues at the smaller districts. We found that the smaller districts were better able to innovate and implement the new technology than the larger districts. This was not necessarily because they were better organized but because they were less burdened by the problems of coordination and communication, problems that tend to increase exponentially with size. Size, however, was not the only factor. Three other important considerations were: (i) management strategies; (ii) management cultures; and (iii) the timing of the implementation process. We have already indicated the role of the managerial culture within each district, enhancing or inhibiting the implementation processes, as well as pointing to the problems of implementing the system at the same time as reorganizing the management structure.

Management strategies and corporate computer systems

Management strategies in the NHS parallel the model set out by Child (1985a), even though these strategies are more policy- than market-driven. Furthermore, they operate within a more pluralistic structure (incorporating medical and nursing hierarchies as well as the managerial) than is typically found within the private sector. Nevertheless, the managerial strategies within the districts were a major influence on the introduction and consequent effects of the corporate computer systems. In large part, these management strategies were concerned with finding ways of coping with the demands of the regional corporate systems policy as much as implementing the systems themselves. One of the major reasons for this qualified enthusiasm for the systems, and in particular MPIS[2], related directly to the timing of the systems' introduction. This conflicted with the demands on districts to establish a new management structure (Griffiths) and install new Körner-inspired information systems. It was also the case that the priorities of district managers had been as much related to their retaining autonomy from direct central control as with utilizing the computer systems to establish integrated management information within their districts.

The management strategies which were the most effective in subordinating the corporate computer systems to the perceived requirements of the district general management, or at least minimize the organizational disruption attendant on the implementation processes, were those of 'corporacy' and 'committed pragmatism'. The first was an overarching proactive strategy of higher management designed to incorporate the interests of all functions and levels of management. The North District seemed to have been able to follow an effective management strategy that was suitable for their organization and reflecting directly the Griffiths general management model. There were, however, qualifications to be made to this assertion with regard to managers of professional and semi-professional staff where the effectiveness of the corporate strategy was attenuated by their countervailing commitment to their own occupational professionalism.

'Committed pragmatism' was the strategy of district managers confronted with the requirement from region to implement a system which was 'out of phase' with existing organizational structures, but which was thought to be a technical prerequisite for the new arrangements being introduced. The result was a pragmatic strategy of getting staff involved in the process of getting the computer system up and running, but delaying any practical consideration as to how it might contribute to the future system of district management.

In contrast, the other strategies either avoided consultation and participation or resulted in little taking place. 'Pragmatic separatism' and 'systems isolationism' were the strategies of those districts where the corporate computer systems had either been implemented in virtual iso-

Figure 10.1 Management strategies, structures and the organizational context

Strategies Systems
    isolationism
      Pragmatism
      • Pragmatic separatism
      • Committed pragmatism

           District corporacy

Structures
Consensus
management ————————————————————▶ General
(1974)

               (1986)

Context
————————▶ Griffiths and
      Körner Reports ————————▶ Regional

Corporate computer policy

lation from the rest of the district organization ('systems isolationism') or the implementation had been undertaken as a simulation exercise by an exclusive steering group of managers and staff who had little opportunity of being able to ascertain whether the procedures adopted would meet the local requirements of other managers and users in the district ('pragmatic separatism'). The rationale for these separatist/isolationist strategies was that they reflected the conditions confronting the larger districts principally, but not entirely, because they were undergoing major reorganizations. The main difference between the two strategies was that *separatism* was intended to facilitate the *formal* implementation of the system while the *isolationist* strategy had as its outcome the *avoidance* of using the system already implemented – because the managers were unconvinced of the value of the system to their informational needs.

The relationship between the four strategies and the organizational context can be diagramatically represented (see Fig. 10.1). This diagram illustrates (in a much simplified form) the temporal relationship between the district management strategies, organizational structures and context, indicating that the strategy of each district had its own logic when considered in light of the conditions prevailing when the systems were first implemented.

We are not suggesting that the strategies were causally determined, only that they can be explained as rational responses to the specific organizational context of regional and DHSS/NHS policies mediated by the organizational arrangements in place within the districts. Change either or both of these and the strategy is likely to alter to bring the districts' policies and action into congruence with the new circumstances. Whether this means that all districts will ultimately develop managerial strategies to match the intended corporate structures of general management we do not know. While the proposed structure of general management favours corporate approaches they will only take root if the managers themselves are convinced of the worth of this innovation to the NHS culture (Harrison, 1986).

Notes

1 These examples are taken from Butler and Vaile (1984), p. 88.
2 The region was to abandon the MPIS system two years later in 1988; the system was never to claim the whole-hearted support of district and unit management and staff.

References

British Journal of Healthcare Computing (1984) Körner implementation gets backing from government, *BJHC*, **1**(2), 5.

Burns, T. (1955) The reference of conduct in small groups: cliques and cabals in occupational milieux. *Human Relations*, **8**, 467–86.

Butler, J.R. and Vaile, E.K. (1984) *Health and Health Services: An Introduction to Health Care in Britain*. London: Routledge and Kegan Paul.

Child, J. (1973) Organisations: a choice for man. In: *Man and Organisation*, Child, J. (ed.). London: George Allen & Unwin.

Child, J. (1985a) Management strategies, new technologies and the labour process. In: *Job Redesign: Critical Perspectives on the Labour Process*, Knights, D. *et al.* (ed.). Aldershot: Gower.

Child, J. (1985b) *Organisation: A Guide to Problems and Practice*, 2nd edn. London: Harper & Row.

Dent, M. (1988) Doctors and Computers. Ph.D. Thesis, University of Warwick.

Griffiths Report (1983) *NHS Management Inquiry*. London: DHSS.

Ham, C. (1985) *Health Policy in Britain*, 2nd edn. London: Macmillan.

Harrison, S. (1986) Management culture and management budgets. *Hospital and Health Service Review*, January, 6–9.

Mason, A. (1984) Körner progress report. *British Journal of Healthcare Computing*, **1**(1), 24–5.

Pettigrew, A. (1979) On studying organizational cultures. *Administrative Science Quarterly*, **24**, pp. 570–81.

Windsor, P. (1984), Editorial; the beginning of the end. *British Journal of Healthcare Computing*, **1**(2), 3.

Appendix 10.1 Organizational size

Number of employees (Full-time equivalents)

South	North	East	West
3516*	2459*	2500**	4321***

Note: Statistics obtained from the district personnel departments: * 1985; ** 1984; *** 1986

*Home population**

South	North	East	West
264 949	175 000	198 100	253 000

* Home population being the basic constituency of the patients

Appendix 10.2 Complexity

	South	*North*	*East*	*West*
Management units	3	3	4	(to be 2 units)
Acute	General*	General	General	General
	Central	Manor		Princess
	Grange	Children's		Eye Hospital
Mental handicap	St Mary's	The Grange	Southdowns	None
	Flower Hill	Hollywell Hall		
Mental illness	*see* Community	*see* Community	Ivy Grange	*see* Community
Community	The Elms	No hospital units	Community unit	Oaktree

* Names have been given to these hospitals in order not to confuse the distinction between 'management unit' and 'hospital unit'. The names however are entirely fictitious
Sources: District Health Authorities Annual Programmes, District Strategy 1985–1994 or by direct communication and correspondence

11 | Innovation and the Politics of Patient Information Systems

Sheri Ahmad

The history of patient information systems in the NHS dates back to the mid-1960s when medium-to-large mainframe systems were commissioned in various regional headquarters, teaching hospitals and specialist computer centres set up by some Regional Health Authorities for experimentation and development of specific software. Noteworthy examples are the development of a Patient Administration System (PAS) by the West Midlands Regional Health Authority in Birmingham in the late 1960s and the batch-processed Accident and Emergency database system introduced by the South Western Regional Health Authority at Bristol in the early 1970s. Laboratory systems, highly specialized and task orientated, were commissioned in the fields of haematology and biochemistry across the country during the mid-1970s. There were also initiatives in the field of pharmacy systems in teaching hospitals to provide information on current prescription of drugs to in-patients and routine and repetitive prescription for patients in general practice.

This chapter focusses on the subject of computerization of medical records in Accident and Emergency (A & E) departments. A brief insight into the workload of an A & E department would be a useful introduction to the case. Nationally one person in five attends an A & E department annually. In 1989 there were just over 11 million such attendances. In order to record a patient's attendance in an A & E department, the reception clerks need to take personal details, the doctor has to record the history, the results of the examination and further investigations together with treatment details; the nurse makes brief notes on the nursing care provided. If the A & E department has a facility to store coded data, the accident officer attending or, rarely, a coding clerk records the information in this form. In the majority of cases an A & E record consists of an

A4-sized card but many other types and sizes exist. Once this record is created and the patient treated, the card is filed for such times as when the patient has a new injury. In an emergency the whole procedure is repeated, resulting in a second card.

Legislation requires that medical records related to an A & E attendance are retained in hard copy form for a period of eight years. This creates a very heavy workload and a departmental responsibility for creating new records, filing and retrieving for re-attendances and, finally, for their accurate storage and retrieval over many years. The sheer nature of A & E work demands a fast, fail-safe retrieval system which almost always means storage within, or very near to, the department. Space has always been at a premium in busy hospitals across the UK. The scope and variety of the activity makes storage a massive problem and consequently retrieval is made difficult and not always successful.

There are other factors that add to the difficulties. A & E departments historically have been treated as the Cinderellas of the NHS. A frequent area of neglect in an average A & E department has been staffing in general and particularly in the reception. Not all A & E departments have 24-hour staffing in this area. Inadequately staffed reception results in poor record creation which, in turn, means poor feedback. If we do not know what is coming through an A & E department we cannot possibly know how best to plan for it. Therefore the importance of having good quality analysis cannot be over-stressed.

Patient information systems – a personal experience

Problem identification

I took up my new appointment as a consultant in an A & E department in an industrial district on 1 January 1979. It was great to start on a day off, oblivious to the problems ahead; I have not had that experience since. I had been used to a very high quality of information, as well as an excellent storage and retrieval system, in my previous hospital. What I inherited as a consultant in charge of my new, and a very busy, A & E department was the 'Lloyd George' envelope type of a card that most GPs still use. It had only five pieces of personal details about a patient, which did not include the patient's sex. The medical records officer who had introduced this card on the day that I commenced work in the new post, on 1 January 1979, was at pains to explain why the sex was omitted. It was to keep the patients from the surrounding factory district from saying 'Yes please' and thus embarrassing the reception staff. To my utter frustration I learnt that a quarter of a million of these cards had been printed and were in storage. My initial appointment to the consultant post had been made the year before, in October 1978, yet the Area Health Authority had not thought it was at all important to seek my opinion on the design of this central tool.

It became clear in my own mind that I needed to computerize the A & E medical records. I set myself four basic objectives:

1 To overcome the storage problem.
2 To make retrieval of records faster and more successful.
3 To be able to write to GPs in each case of attendance at the A & E department.
4 To have a statistical feedback.

It did not take very long to find out that in 1979 such a computerized information system did not exist in the UK. If one needed it badly it had to be created. The idea of a system which would be all things for an A & E service was attractive but it needed approval from various quarters. There were four main groups who had to accept the concept before progress could be made. They were doctors, nurses, the medical secretariat, clerical staff and of course the administrators (but not necessarily in this order). I discussed the subject in principle with my peer group and especially the casualty surgeons in the Region. It was extremely encouraging to learn that there was whole-hearted support from all the A & E consultants and especially from my working partner who was in charge of the A & E department at the other major district hospital. I then took the idea informally to the District Administrator and the District Medical Officer and found both of them receptive. However, they needed to see a firm proposal and a formal presentation to the District Management Team. Before I could proceed any further it was necessary to test out the idea among the secretaries, receptionists, medical records officers and nurses.

Finding local solutions

This is where I started to encounter widely differing reactions. The main underlying fears were of change and technology. The word 'computer' was familiar but 'computer technology' was new in this context and the expression 'information technology' had not been heard of. I had started my job with only a part-time secretary, not an uncommon phenomenon in the NHS where new consultant posts are not always supported and therefore never fully productive from day one. Her half life to me came to a sudden decay on hearing the word 'computer'. The same thing happened to the second half that was arranged for me. On reflection over the years, both the halves belonged to ladies who were well established in their careers and had no wish to learn new tricks. Those early months gave me a valuable first-hand experience which was to re-shape my approach later.

The reception staff did not think that my ideas about medical records were at all practical. Their feeling was that it would never work. The nurses were very interested as long as they did not have to do anything extra. It was strange to me that this group of colleagues wished to make no input nor derive anything from it. To this day I have discovered no answer as to why this was so.

While all this was being talked about I was also increasingly puzzled because Medical Record Officers in the hospital administration neither took to the idea nor resisted it. I had expected a considerable reaction to what was essentially invasion of their work environment. Further knowledge and experience reinforced my earlier belief that A & E departments are neglected or under-supported within the NHS. Those responsible for medical records nationally have not generally taken a keen and active interest in their A & E records. There are many reasons for this. Firstly A & E records' activity is largely an independent, intensive and self-contained 24-hour segment within the medical records' service to a hospital or a district. In their isolation staff sometimes tend to develop anti-social attitudes. Generally there are two types of people found in the A & E reception. There are those who like the high pressure and socially demanding environment which brings them to the forefront of patient encounters. They are there by choice. They form a vital part of an A & E team and I consider them one of the three pillars of the service. The other type are those who were sent there for various reasons by their masters. This type do a mediocre job and remain unhappy and find it difficult to team up with the A & E doctors and nurses.

More importantly perhaps, central records tend to place emphasis on the flow of patients in and out of hospital beds and to leave A & E records to people on the spot. This view accords well with the priorities of the most influential practitioners. In these circumstances one needs to strengthen the A & E clerical structure to a level that they perform as an independent, dedicated team. Rotas that require interchange between A & E reception staff and the central hospital medical records clerks lead to poor service. They are two very different kinds of people fulfilling very different roles. It is like expecting the assembly line workers from a bicycle factory to change places with their counterparts in a motor car industry and vice versa. I therefore sought reassurance from the administration and medical records officers that there should be a 24-hour staffing in the A & E reception and that the staff would work, as far as possible, as an independent team. At about the same time, a survey carried out by the administration showed that the work load was such that I needed three full-time secretaries and a similar number for my working partner in the other A & E department.

We made an initial proposal to computerize the A & E records in April 1979 and soon after a demonstration of a possible solution. Both the presentations were well received by the Area and District administration. This experiment followed a very long and arduous process in which my proposal had been presented at meetings, committees and informal discussions at District, Area and Regional levels of administration. Finally the Regional Health Authority kindly agreed to fund three systems to be put into the following:

1 The District general hospital where I was based.
2 A second District general hospital where my partner was based.

3 A general hospital in another District where a senior colleague of ours
  was based. (He had put up his own proposal for a computerized records
  system some four years earlier in 1975 without success.)

Designing and implementing the project

I then started the process of discussions with the Management Services
Department at the Regional Health Authority to prepare a tender document. This was a frustrating phase and took many months. However, at
each administrative bottle neck I was helped by the senior officers both at
the Region and the District Health Authority. It took about 20 months
from agreement in principle for the Regional Health Authority to fund
three systems to the time when invitations to tender on price were sent
out. In the meantime a third of the money had been withdrawn by the
Regional Health Authority so that only two systems could be purchased.
We had a gentleman's agreement that our District should have one and the
other District the second, but each of the districts had to accept the
running costs. In our District Health Authority, the Senior Officer was a
keen sponsor of my idea so that there was no difficulty in the Authority
accepting the running costs. Our system based on an IBM System 6
information processor was delivered to my hospital in March 1981. The
story in the other District was different. Their programme continued to
slip and in 1982 all hope was given up.

Implementation of the first 'pilot system' at my hospital took almost
two years. Difficulties encountered in installation, simple things like
power points and lighting took months to have changed. Recruitment of a
new supervisor and replacement of the secretaries that had resigned was
augmented by time taken in their training. There was considerable resistance to change among the reception staff which made training into and
adaptation of the system extremely time-consuming. By the early part of
1983 the system was fully implemented. The lessons learnt were written
up as a systems review report and a paper was presented at the International Medical Informatics Conference at Dublin in 1982.

Adaptation and diffusion

By this time a new District general hospital for our District was slowly
nearing completion. It had been agreed that the two A & E departments,
the one at my hospital and the other at the second general hospital would
be closed to new patients and that the A & E department at the new
hospital would take all new patients. We were quite concerned as to how
that would be possible because the combined totals of the two A & E
departments were far greater than the planned total for which the new
department had been designed. The administrators' attitude was that not
all the people who used the previous two departments would like to travel

to the new hospital and it was their hope that some potential patients would go to the neighbouring districts in future. I was sceptical about this.

Among other things we were asked what system of record keeping we would want at the new A & E department. I had learnt a lot from the pilot system at the previous hospital and I was ready to design an improved system for the new A & E department. However, informal discussions with all colleagues in the Region led us to believe that there was support for a common system in the Region. I had presented a paper entitled 'The way forward in accident and emergency record keeping' at the Casualty Surgeons Association (CSA) Annual Conference of 1982 which was later published in the *British Journal of Accident and Emergency Medicine*. The points made in the paper formed the basis for discussion among the 15 or so consultants in A & E in the Region at the time.

We held a one-day workshop attended by all consultants, senior registrars and registrars in A & E, a few invited administrators, medical record officers and some medical secretaries. The database, system of coding, the text input, system features and letters were discussed and agreed. A second session attended by four nominated consultants agreed a system of ICD coding for A & E work. Based on the agreed parameters and features, I wrote a system specification which was submitted to the Regional Health Authority for acceptance as a standard system for A & E departments in the Region. The senior officers at District Health Authority and at the Region level were once again very keen on the idea and, indeed, were my strongest sponsors.

However, the proposal continued to encounter the strongest opposition from the computer specialists in the Management Services Department of the Regional Health Authority. A number of hurdles were created for us by their requests for fuller information but the absolute pit was their insistence that we should choose the hardware from a manufacturer that the Region had experience of and with whom the Authority had preferential purchase agreements. We were told that not only would we have to have a Model T Ford but that we could have it only in black. The reasons for this stance derived from the needs of the Regional Standards System. I was in fact very open minded about the discussion of hardware. I maintained that we knew all about the Model T in black and it was not going to be our carriage, but that we would consider anything out of the remaining 99 manufacturers. Under such circumstances, I was made to understand, there would be no progress. I had obviously failed to get the message and therefore continued in my optimistic belief that logic would prevail. It was not to be an easy time ahead.

At this stage we were asked to present the case to the Regional Information Systems Committee (RISC) in order to obtain agreement for the allocation of money and a go-ahead to tender. I attended a meeting of the RISC together with two very good officers from Management Services who had been assigned to the project in order to help in the preparation of our case. The membership of RISC in attendance that afternoon was between 12 and 14 in spite of the generally erratic comings and goings of its membership. Against that number a single spokesman helped by two officers had to present a case for the practitioners against that put forward by the experts in Management Services who advised RISC.

We were given half an hour on the agenda. In actual fact it took over two hours out of my life in the most painful and utterly useless game play. I finally picked up my jacket, papers and pointer and, closely followed by my two minders, proceeded to leave the meeting. One dedicated player shouted after me wishing to know where I would get the money for the project without their consent. My reply to this question, unique in the history of an NHS committee, has been repeated many times by others in telling the story.

I returned home directly because I was too angry and frustrated to do anything useful. It was a bright summer evening and in order to calm down I mowed the lawns, front and back, something I had hardly ever done, and still I was angry. I was later to recall this meeting many times and could never find justification for the time wasted by some 16–17 highly paid officers. I can still see the doodles being drawn by many people around the table. Some, large, dark and very elaborate, indicated their totally detached minds, while others drew small frustrated symbols. One character, who had had the best of the sandwiches and dessert earlier, remained fast asleep throughout. The chairman of the committee was the only person trying hard to make some sense out of the afternoon. During the course of the meeting he asked permission of the members to make a statement aside from the chair in an expression of his own frustration at their behaviour. I remember well the directness of his analysis but again cannot quote his words.

The following day I reported the lack of progress to my District Administrator and after a brief exchange on his advice rang the Regional Administrator and reported the same. I also conveyed my opinion that he could safely dismantle RISC and matters could only improve. He was sympathetic and encouraging and promised to come back to me within 48 hours. This he did with a few hours to spare and I was overjoyed to hear that we had the money for the project and could proceed at full speed. The tendering process could be put into action immediately as the supplies department had already been informed by him.

The tendering process is a separate story and is, perhaps another insight into why the NHS, at its best, only just grinds ahead. At the conclusion of the tendering process the necessary contracts were awarded to my chosen IBM hardware and software firm. The successful combination of hardware and software firms gave a solution well within a budget of £250 000 for two systems, one at our new District hospital and the other at the neighbouring District that had failed on two previous occasions. The software was to be written to our specification and later it was planned to adapt this software to communicate interactively with the hospital's ICL-based PAS. Completion for the whole project was to be within six months. This compared with the alternative solution that had been put forward by the experts in Management Services which was estimated at over £350 000 and would have taken about three years to complete. Their solution was mainframe based and had considerable knock-on effects in building work, air conditioning, extra staff and hence much higher revenue consequences as well.

The hardware, an IBM System 36, containing 15 VDUs, three printers, a PC and six colour plotters was delivered to our A & E department in December 1984. It was plugged into the existing power supply in a room which had been set aside for the system and within days the system was configured through the cabling which had been put in very efficiently by a local firm only weeks before.

Then started our next period of waste and frustration. Before the software firm could start to write the software, which was to be in RPG11, they had to submit the system specification for approval by the Regional Health Authority. This was announced rather suddenly by the Regional Health Authority representative in the local steering group that had been set up to implement the project. Further questions elicited a reply that what I had written was an outline system specification which now had to be converted to a technical specification for approval by the Management Services Department. The group of officers who had responsibility for the development of the Regional Standards System (RSS) for the ICL-based PAS in the new hospital were the only people who could ensure that our A & E system would be compatible with the latter and therefore capable of interactive communication.

This was 'management-speak', but to all the clinicians in the steering group it meant one thing – delays. To make matters worse, the two officers assigned to the project by the Management Services Department had to leave. Both of them were bright and had put in more than an honest day's work. They had also worked without bias or prejudice. One of them applied for a higher grade job in a neighbouring District and very deservedly got it. The second person was moved to another job within the Region. Their replacements appeared more aware of the Management Services Department's hostility towards the project. Their coming co-incided with two other changes in the steering group membership. There then followed nine months of highly acrimonious and wasteful meetings: on one occasion legal action was threatened. But the familiar tactics of the Management Services Department's representatives were not to turn up for a meeting or to ring the secretary one week before the meeting and ask for a change in the date. The actual work required to produce the technical specification could have been comfortably completed in less than three weeks. In fact the total number of hours worked were less than even that, but the time actually taken over this phase was nine months.

The actual writing of software was completed within a matter of weeks. One team leader was an external systems consultant and author of the software. He displayed an exceptional mind in replying to speeches made by the Management Services Department's personnel with replies in single lines or short phrases. His work represented his true eloquence in RPG11 protocols. His expertise became increasingly obvious in the testing and acceptance stage which was completed within a few weeks.

The system went operational at the most basic level (1) on 3 June 1986. Levels of increasing sophistication (2 and 3) were achieved within the year. The ultimate test of the system at technical, practical and human levels came through the experiences of all those who used it and came to rely on it from those different angles. It is now four years old and it has not gone down once, or lost a file, except through human error, or slowed down. The receptionists, secretaries, nurses (who originally wished not to have anything to do with it) and doctors have come to depend on it absolutely. It is a truly user–affectionate system.

More importantly, the care of our patients has been made very much easier and better. The GPs are kept informed in detail of every patient that attends the A & E department at Russells Hall which is now the busiest in the country. Since commissioning the system our quarter of a millionth attendance was achieved early in 1988. Over that time it had picked up suspected cases of non–accidental injuries (NAI) before serious harm had been done to children at risk in their domestic environment. It provides a sub–second response to a search and reproduction of a single record out of a possible 400000 which enables all kinds of new analyses of data to be undertaken. It has made it easier for us to manage the known sufferers – a category which includes asthmatics, diabetics, brittle bones, epileptics, hospital hoppers (itinerant hypochondriacs), drug addicts, patients on anti-coagulants, haemophiliacs and, more lately, AIDS sufferers. It has also given extremely useful feedback on the development of allergies that have been previously recorded. Through the valuable clinical management information that it has provided it has changed the way we work. Based on this information our staffing patterns have been changed for the benefit of the patients.

Implications for the NHS

The same benefits could be derived from the application of information technology to the rest of the A & E services in the country if the administrative and clinical prejudices could be overcome. It is possible today to produce the injury profile of the whole nation and to initiate appropriate preventative measures. Any kind of injury or combination of features related to such injury can be studied and analysed in much greater detail than ever before. Case analysis can be attempted when there is scant information available.

The UK NHS still remains the finest health service in the world. In 1988 I visited several A & E departments in high-density population areas as well as centres of excellence, in the USA, Japan and China. I was quietly pleased to discover that a good A & E department in the UK provides better overall services to the patient attending than anywhere else in the world. However, the NHS has always had the momentum of a super tanker. It is always difficult to get under way and once moving extremely slow to turn or make a stop. The Griffiths reorganization has meant an overnight refit to add fins, trim-tabs and hydrofoils. The reader can draw their own conclusions on its present performance. It is unimaginable that by simply changing the labels from administrators to managers the performance would improve. Several years after the attempted reorganization, management remains exercised largely on the basis of complaint and savings are incurred through neglect.

In this extremely elaborate bureaucracy certain tendencies to self-destruction emerge. I will discuss them briefly. The time it takes in the NHS from conception of an idea, through planning to implementation is now always longer than the useful life of the idea. Obsolescence is built into the system. The state of neglect that exists in the NHS, whether it is buildings, equipment or routine practices, has no parallel in private or corporate industry. The increasing chaos in neglected areas can be explained by the Second Law of Thermodynamics. This states that the entropy or disorder of a system always increases with time.

One small example from A & E procedures illustrates the point very well. When a patient is discharged from the hospital having received treatment, details should be sent to his or her GP. A GP who has not heard from the hospital as to what was done to the patient will in urgent matters telephone the hospital for some information. Such calls are usually routed, in the first instance, to the central medical records officer and eventually will end up with the medical secretary to the consultant. The secretary in turn may have to leave her desk to look for the patient's records retained locally and even then can only answer some of the questions. Often enough, medical staff or the consultant in charge of the case has eventually to handle the call. This process usually takes place between 9.00 a.m. and 5.00 p.m., but more often during morning surgery hours so that considerable time is wasted and telephone bills incurred while each stage of the search proceeds. In procedures adopted within the computerized system described above a letter to the GP is printed automatically. In an electronically networked system the GP's records could be accessed and amended automatically and, if necessary, the dialogue between hospital and the primary carers continued throughout the case life of the patient. In the absence of such a dialogue, the A & E records can be immediately accessed by the medical records clerk on receipt of a GP's telephone call and the necessary information conveyed from the VDU screen or printed out in letter/report form.

The prejudice and political process that continue to delay the introduction of information technology in the NHS is perhaps the biggest hurdle to administrative and clinical progress. For any problem there is a political solution or a logical solution but it is more likely that in the NHS today the choice will be the former rather than the latter. Present political structures allow personalities and personal preferences to shape strategy at all levels. A majority decision in a steering group means little if the key person responsible for its activation does not either like it or worse still has no first-hand knowledge to appreciate or apply it. Many dozens of administrators possess a knowledge of computers that is confined to a particular combination of a certain hardware, operating protocol and language with which they have worked in one environment for more years than they would care to admit. This group have neither kept up with current reading nor the rapid advances made in information technology. It is like an audiophile continuing to play the 78 r.p.m. and fervently believing that His Master's Voice will tell him if there is anything better. The information technology initiative, much encouraged by Mrs Thatcher, with the complementary attempt to improve information systems in the NHS, is floundering. Practitioners are far from having sufficient basic reliable information to operate reflectively day to day. Yet, the technology is available, that with a visionary's application, can solve many of the monumental problems of the NHS with half of today's staff.

12 | Hospitals in the UK: A History of Design Innovation

Gary Vann-Wye

Introduction

This chapter examines the emergence of hospital design in the UK during the latter half of the 20th century. From an initial consideration of the historical background to current hospital design, the chapter passes to an examination of political and economic factors that have shaped design and work organization. The year 1974 proved to be a crucial watershed for health care planning. Indeed the reverberations of the economic crisis signalled in that year can still be felt throughout the service. Consequently this work gives some emphasis to the factors operating in the mid-1970s which fundamentally reshaped ideas of appropriate design responses.

Origins and development of hospital plan-forms, work systems and the nature of template knowledge

The design of a new institutional type leans heavily upon existing exemplars both in terms of physical form and work organization. New types of enterprise adapt existing design formulations developed in other circumstances to their own needs. Existing 'knowledge bases' form 'templates' which act as springboards for action. Legitimacy is thus established through reference to current practice. These organizationally located design *Gestalten* also relate to preferred configurations of resource disposition and work practice, together with customary patterns of hierarchical organization and authority relationships (Kuhn, 1962; Schutz, 1972; Merton, 1973; Alexander 1979).

To understand the evolution of the hospital as a building and organizational type is thus to look at its antecedents. It is also necessary to examine the way in which organizational knowledge and politics work upon established templates or exemplary forms to negotiate new patterns of resource distribution within the process of design/redesign.

Pre-industrial forms

The church and religious orders. Care of the sick was regarded as an expression of the Christian virtue of charity. Its development upon an organized basis within the religious orders introduced several elements which were to become characteristic of hospital care. These included the adaptation of the Roman Basilican church plan-form as the basis for the hospital ward. Certain other features such as the uniformed care of the sick, an hierarchical authority structure, and segregation from the outside world followed directly from the traditions of monastic life. Furthermore, the establishment of a 'priesthood' of specialist practitioners laid the foundations for the later dominance of an elite medical profession. In some cases church and military influence combined, as in the work of the Knights of St John, who were amongst the first to establish reporting, record keeping and the separation of nursing and medical functions.

The military. Military medical practice has exerted a profound influence upon civilian hospital care. The treatment of large numbers of battlefield casualties under field conditions encouraged the development of command systems deriving from the organization of battle itself. The present-day perception of health care as an acute curative service owes much to this ancestry. The high prestige of accident and emergency services amongst the working staffs of UK hospitals preserves the early model of medicine as a disciplined mechanism confronting natural and man-made disaster. The use of particular techniques of discipline and surveillance as part of the military ethos left a definite stamp upon the physical design and authority structures of hospitals. Hospital buildings were viewed as disciplinary mechanisms with each separate functional activity connected with a system of patient inspection, evaluation and control (Foucault, 1977).

The penal system. Prisons and hospitals share certain basic design problems. These include the confinement and control of a large and potentially hazardous clientele. There is a need for observation, segregation and regulated contact with the external social world. At several points during the history of hospital and prison design development there was a mutual infusion of design ideals between the two types. The custodial dimensions of thought incorporated in hospital layouts are well evidenced in projects such as Bentham's 'Panopticon', whose therapeutic efficacy was thought to be equally suited to clinical and penal purposes (Foucault, 1977).

The poor-house. The institution of housing for the poor had its roots in the accommodation provided for the unfortunate and impecunious by religious, civil and charitable bodies. The term 'hospital' was originally a designation applied to almshouses for the parish poor. The almshouse advanced the opposite plan type to that of the military barrack room, featuring cubicled dwelling spaces around a courtyard or cloister layout. The development of these smaller units into the workhouse system in the 18th and 19th centuries represented an effort to regulate the distribution of relief to the poor, the old and the infirm. The adaptation of workhouse ideals in charity hospitals aimed at discovering malingerers and at moral reform in addition to medical treatment. The regime of sobriety and discipline applied to the workhouse population provided a model for hospitals dealing with the lower orders (Forty, 1980).

The factory. The factory system introduced several features into patterns of employment which fed into the development of hospital-based health care. Significant amongst these were continuous working, the shift system, the use of capital-intensive equipment to process raw materials, the centralization of production to reduce cost and to monopolize the provision of goods and services. These industrial influences found their way into hospitals from the 18th century onwards. That they did so is all the more surprising given a tradition of professional self-identification which stressed patient-centredness. Hospital staff did not, and still do not, see hospitals as industrial enterprises, but factory culture has had a profound effect upon labour organization. Penetration of industrial value has, however, not been uniform. Those elements of hospital work systems not protected from managerialist encroachment such as portering, cleaning and catering have become the first to be subject to work measurement and proletarianization.

The English country house. An important architectural template for late 18th and 19th century hospitals was that of the country house. The use of Palladian and other forms of Neo-Classical façades furnished a visual rhetoric which attracted philanthropy and voluntary subscription. Benefactors could gain status by supporting projects which aped fashionable taste, and achieve upward mobility by associating with aristocratic patrons of hospital developments. The country house contributed a further design element: that of a cordon sanitaire. The erection of hospital buildings on country sites not only gave them a separate and distinct institutional character, but came to be supported by Florence Nightingale and other influential designers as a positive factor in disease control.

The internal planning of these imposing edifices was adapted to the authority patterns of the time. The use of corridors served to reflect the need to insulate different levels of the medical, paramedical and domestic hierarchy (Forty, 1980).

Industrial forms. During the pre-industrial era the first four of the above models proved the most influential. The adoption of ideas for the plan-form of hospitals from these exemplary types combined with their hierarchical and authoritarian control structures to produce a type of institution which put the surveillance of patients and staff high upon its list of priorities. With the rise of urban populations in the 18th and 19th centuries, existing small hospitals became inadequate. Private health care for the well-to-do was usually conducted in the home by independent medical practitioners. Hospital premises were required to house the poor and exercise physical and moral restraint over them during their hospital stay. But the varied ancestry of UK hospitals has already become apparent. These diverse ideas were first codified by the nursing pioneer Florence Nightingale. Nightingale's approach combined philanthropy and public welfare concerns with practical experience of hospital administration gained under field conditions with the British Army and research undertaken by her thereafter. To disseminate her work she drew upon an influential circle of social and political contacts. She was a protagonist of statistical methods, and brought a numerical precision to the specification of building elements. She advocated the pavilion plan in which large open wards accommodating 32 patients were connected by a corridor system. Hospital administration areas, 'hotel services', treatment rooms were separated out as discrete physical territories (Nightingale, 1864). Her contribution to the development of hospital design philosophies was threefold.

- She produced a standard plan type which articulated with some of the most fruitful medical and nursing developments of the time.
- She provided a layout which separated out potentially rival professional groups.
- By the advocacy of a system of large open wards policed by nursing sisters she ensured that the emerging profession of nursing would have uncontested direction over the largest portion of hospital premises.

Nightingale's miasmic conceptions of disease were to be replaced by later formulations but her plan-form proved capable of piecemeal addition and adaptation to house new medical and paramedical specialisms as they arose. Her ideas spread to countries throughout the British Empire and North America. The Nightingale ward left an indelible imprint upon hospital design practice up to the present time. In 1977 there were 2655 hospitals with 463 000 allocated beds within the NHS. Nearly half of these hospitals were built before 1891 (McFarlane *et al.*, 1980). The sheer bulk of hospitals erected in the heyday of Nightingale ideals means that the influence of her design template has remained strong. Although her intentions were not to industrialize hospital care, the approach to design that she pioneered offered several possibilities for rationalizing design and constructional methods.

- By simplifying hospital layouts into separate treatment areas and wards she encouraged the trend towards task specialization and the growth of a style of departmental organization that could adopt and adapt capital intensive treatment techniques. The separation of different specialist areas adopted in her plan enabled the sequential insertion of developing medical technologies without major disruption of physical planning.
- By 'modularizing' ward and other hospital functions within a defined system of dimensioning she pointed the way for the later adoption of standard designs and industrialized building techniques. The Nightingale template demystified hospital design and provided a shared physical and organizational design vocabulary which could be, and to a certain extent was, drawn upon a century later when the Ministry of Health (later DHSS) began to devise a common design database for a state financed service.

The subsequent history of health care in the UK was not, however, to follow a philosophy of industrial organization. The continuing prominence of professional ideology and control over managerialism ensured the rejection of a health care provision based upon factory production and the patterns of unitary control which that has generally been taken to imply.

Welfarism and professionalism. The incorporation of health care as part of a nationally directed programme of social welfare had its roots in the late 19th and early 20th centuries. Connecting with developing concerns for health and safety in the workplace and the need for an efficient workforce, it became a major feature of post-World War II Labour Party policy. War conditions had of themselves created some of the necessary administrative reforms for the establishment of a national health care programme. The founding of the Emergency Medical Service had meant government direction of medical staff and hospital resources. Furthermore it had revealed that the hospital stock and building provision were inadequate, maldistributed and outdated. Abel-Smith notes that under the voluntary system the country had become 'littered with small hospitals'. With the outbreak of World War II (Abel-Smith, 1964, p. 406):

> ... it was found that of about 77 general hospitals only some seventy-five were equipped with over 200 beds, some 115 provided between 100 and 200 beds, over 500 had less than 100 beds, and more than half of these had less than 30 beds.

The siting of most of these units was due to an eccentric combination of factors which included historical accident, charitable intentions, and municipal pride.

It was upon this peculiar physical resource base that projections of a socialized health service had to be erected. To construct a system of delivery that was marked by efficiency and equity was a difficult task, given that charity and local initiative had already created a network marked by strong regional imbalances.

The post-War governments' intentions for the NHS are summarized in Bevan (1976) and the long and protracted bargaining which created the service chronicled in Foot (1973). Although the NHS embodied state funding to provide a service free at the point of delivery, effective control passed to senior medical interests. Government was only to condition the overall size of the health budget. Within the service detailed design of hospital provision, medical technologies, and service distribution was to remain largely a professional affair. In return for policing a state system of sickness and welfare benefits medicine was given a virtually free hand to determine its own internal self-development. The framework of Regional Health Boards and Hospital Management Committees which was created in 1947 gave medical groups strong influence over health care planning at all levels.

The tradition of individualistic professional self-advancement which characterized pre-State control was to continue as the driving force behind the politics of redesign. These forces situated themselves neatly within a socialized employment system which stressed employee participation and humane working conditions. Some, however, achieved more participation than others.

This should not obscure the fact that medical involvement in hospital design came fairly late in the day. Not until the last quarter of the 19th century did hospital design attract medical interest. Only when the possibility of using hospital patients as raw material in the development of a 'scientific' rationale for medicine was recognized did active medical participation in hospital designing become regarded as important.

The emergence of new forms. Following upon World War II there was no blueprint of what form an NHS hospital should take. What did exist as an established model for development was a pattern of localized private, voluntary and local authority sector initiatives which employed incremental adaptation as a change dynamic. This localized/pluralist mode of design development was to continue. Few new hospitals were built until the early 1960s, but there were important research and design inputs during the 1950s. Continental experiments, especially in the social democratic states of Scandinavia provided an inspiration for the ethos of NHS planning.

One of the most important foundations for the direction of future design work was laid by the Nuffield Foundation's Division of Architectural Studies headed by Richard Llewelyn Davis (Nuffield Trust, 1955). The research team compared conventional Nightingale layouts with variations of the 'corridor' or 'bay' ward arrangement drawn from English, French, Swedish and US designs. The imprint of private medical care with its hotel-type services is clear. The Nuffield study's conclusions incorporated an advocacy of wards consisting of small bays rather than the continued use of open layouts. The researchers employed findings from time and motion studies made of tasks and staff circulation in wards (Nuffield Trust, 1955). This research was used to underpin an attack upon the prevailing belief that open wards were more efficient in terms of the use of staff time. The Nuffield designers recommended the provision of treatment and ancillary rooms in ward units. Wards were to be as large as practicable to economize on administration. A further significant feature of the Nuffield study was its treatment of the technical requirements of hospitals which pointed the way to the establishment of an organized data base by the DHSS.

However, the mid- and late-1950s were a time of groping towards possible new configurations of the design of NHS hospitals. Noakes (1982) has dubbed this post-war period as one of 'make do and mend' where Ministry of Health architects confined themselves to projects which largely consisted of the refurbishment of existing buildings. A lack of clarity of aims and intentions was present at the highest levels of the NHS design hierarchy. In 1960 an important exhibition and conference was held by the Royal Institute of British Architects as an attempt to clarify conceptions of the way forward.

Contributors to the conference were divided on whether hospitals should be planned as 'one offs' peculiar to each site or whether standardized planning was desirable. However, there was an underlying belief in architectural and design circles that technical studies and a functionalist design philosophy would lead to solutions. This belief in functionalist solutions and systematic research was to take root in the Department of Health. In 1958 Tatton Brown became the first Ministry of Health Chief Architect. His experience in school design and industrialized building techniques was a spur for the first series of 'Departmental Hospital Building and Equipment Notes and Technical Memoranda' aimed at promoting good practice and codification of standards.

Despite these early attempts at coordination of design work and the setting of parameters for levels of provision the precise form of NHS hospitals was still an open question in the early 1960s. The 'Hospital Plan for England and Wales' (1962) went some way towards setting a specification for the overall shape of the NHS hospital service. It attempted to define building needs and to project building project starts for a period of ten years. Taking population estimates it laid down bed ratios for different medical specialisms. The plan stipulated how the numbers of beds and out-patient facilities should be grouped and distributed. The key concept was that of the 'District General Hospital' (DGH). The Ministry's DGH philosophy took its justification from a claimed interdependence of different branches of medicine and the need to bring together a range of core facilities for diagnosis and treatment. This conception implied that for a viable hospital unit a certain minimal 'chunk' of resources was required. Rival hospital forms such as specialist clinics, cottage hospitals and community-based care options were defined as unsatisfactory. The optimal size of the DGH was 600–800 beds serving a population of 100 000 to 150 000. Regional specialities requiring larger catchment areas would be provided at selected centres. As the DGH network grew, smaller hospitals would be closed.

Within the prevailing climate of architectural experiment in hospital design the imposition of the overall 'Hospital Plan' had few immediate effects on unit standardization. Regional authorities and their private architectural consultants regarded hospital designing as a creative one-off process. Departmental advice was regarded as just that, there was little indication of uniform planning (Gainsborough and Gainsborough, 1964). Local and intra-organizational interests, different practitioner preferences and bodies external to the NHS fed in decisive ideas on design. But these variations culminated in the development of distinct regional design models such as the 'Oxford' and 'Birmingham' methods. These incorporate earlier innovations such as the cubicled ward, but were to create significant differences in layout.

In the emerging contest between regions, the Ministry of Health attempted to attain a lead with a series of small-scale development projects concentrating upon departmental design. Those at Walton Hospital (Liverpool) and Kingston Hospital (Surrey) sought to test out new cost control systems developed from 'Departmental Building Notes'. These piecemeal attempts were followed by a whole hospital project at Greenwich Hospital commenced in 1962. Holroyd (1968) noted its similarity to Palo Alto Hospital in the USA. The building of its UK counterpart was eventually completed in 1976. Green (1971) saw the project as epitomizing a growing separation between physical design and 'functionalism' in work design. This lack of integration in physical planning and work organization was later to be noted by Vann-Wye (1986) and by Grieco (see Chapter 14). Both authors report widely differing systems of work organization within a standard physical layout in spite of their intended complementarity. The reason derives from the relative influence exercised by the professional interest groups involved in the commissioning stages and in later incremental adaptations to work practice within the completed hospital shell (see also Sharifi, Chapter 13).

The pursuit of rationalism

In 1966 the Ministry of Health admitted that their projected building programme had timescales that were too short and catered for a population that was too small. The UK's lagging economic performance was causing the Government to look hard at the cost of new hospital building. The 'Best Buy' design, commenced in 1967, was a departmental response to the new mode of stringency. Cost cutting was achieved by assuming greater dependence upon community-based services, reduction of bed ratios for acute medical and surgical specialities from 3 to 2 per 1000, and by adoption of policies of earlier discharge. 'Best Buy' was seen as a minimum specification hospital and its cost saving advantage summed up in the slogan 'two for the price of one'. The design incorporated the Central Treatment Area (CTA) concept which sought to increase the throughput of day surgery work.

Cost savings were certainly achieved through the use of the 'Best Buy' format (DHSS/COI, 1973). But 'Best Buy' does not seem to have been a deliberate attempt by central government to impose uniform planning solutions. It became a 'standard' design by default as funding difficulties began to invalidate 'one-off' design approaches. The late 1960s saw a reversal of financial circumstances. Against this newly optimistic economic background the DHSS conceived 'Harness' – a detailed and costly standard design solution using computer-aided design (CAD) and incorporating the recommendations for centrally integrated services set forth in the Bonham Carter Report (1969).

'Harness', developed in conjunction with several Regional Health Authorities, represented a high point in departmental attempts at standardization. It sought to produce complete document packages to contractors. The design envisaged drastic reductions in hospital planning periods. It projected hospitals of 600–1000 beds and was lavish in providing generous levels of accommodation. With 'Harness' visions of the high-tech super DGH had come of age. The involvement of Regions in the design's development forestalled any suggestions of centrally imposed standards.

Several events led to the design's rapid demise. Projects ran into construction problems and there were criticisms of wasted space and of the over-loose fit of the 'Harness' building envelope (James, 1974; O'Neill, 1980). Most serious of all, the 1974 recession made the continuance of its highly costly provisions impossible to maintain. Dudley and Stafford hospitals were the only two major schemes completed, along with four other minor projects.

The outcome of the new economic scenario was the development of a stripped first phase hospital design solution called 'Nucleus'. Although 'Best Buy' had been a cheap solution it proved unsuitable. It was conceived as a whole hospital design and thus too expensive to build in one chunk given the post-1974 cutbacks. 'Nucleus' was based upon the idea of phased development – a minimum viable first-phase development capable of receiving later additions.

The work on 'Nucleus' took place under very adverse conditions. The DHSS was in the throes of the 1974 reorganization and the design teams assembled under the 'Harness' programme had been disbanded. A design had to be developed quickly and this meant a centrally devised solution assembled without the customary consultation procedures. Geoff Mayers, one of the DHSS officers involved, commented later (*Health and Social Services Journal*, 1979, p. 336): 'We came up with the initial idea of a "Nucleus" hospital virtually within a week.'

Time was saved by adapting the 'Harness' template and cutting down the levels of provision. By 1978 the DHSS had produced layouts for a basic range of hospitals distributed to health authorities as a design library. Internal NHS developments had made adherence to the emerging 'Nucleus' concepts more pressing. The Minister, himself a former medical practitioner, argued for 'Nucleus', and pointed out the lack of standard design practice within the service had resulted in costly delays. However, the truncation of the customary consultations with medical interests led to attacks upon the Ministry in the medical press (for example, *British Medical Journal*, 31 January 1976, pp. 245–6).

The design philosophy was summarized in the DHSS document *Nucleus* (1976). The intention was to provide an extendable first-phase development with priority given to economy in capital and running costs. Engineering services provided were sufficient only for the accommodation built. Multi-use of space was envisaged and this latter idea embodied a threat to existing forms of hospital territorial segregation. In many ways 'Nucleus' represented a return to the pavilion layouts beloved of Nightingale. Ward and departmental cruciform templates were strung together by the use of a hospital street. Yet traditional territorial boundaries were preserved – just. The use of light partitioning within the cruciform planning modules was intended to allow rapid re-design of a hospital in use. There was the possibility of quickly altering the relationships between department areas and re-allocating space as needs changed. In practice, this flexibility was to be limited by the involvement of senior hospital staff at the Area (later District) level of implementation who acted to restore permanency to territorial boundaries.

Initially the DHSS had some success in imposing its ideals upon some health authorities. In the early 'Nucleus' developments, departmental offices seemed to have taken a strong line on the integrity of the design solution. Detailed case study evidence (Vann-Wye, 1986) supports the view that there was strong pressure from the centre to enforce design control upon Regional and Area authorities in the mid- to late-1970s. But within the complex political processes of the NHS, local interests sought to modify the 'Nucleus' code. The DHSS found it impossible to enforce a uniform design system. By early 1979 there was official recognition of the wide range of deviations from 'standard Nucleus' design material.

Notwithstanding this the 'Nucleus' guidelines had more success than any previous post-War template. The tightness of NHS finance had made the enforcement of 'Nucleus' space standards more effective than most health authorities would have liked. In September 1980 a conference on 'Nucleus' at the King Edward's Hospital Fund Centre saw widespread complaints of the 'tyranny' of the 'Nucleus' blueprint (King Edward's Hospital Fund Centre, 1981). At this time 40 'Nucleus' schemes were under way and the first prototype had been completed. At a later conference in January 1981 'Nucleus' again came under criticism and a study by the Worcester Health Authority (Checkletts *et al.*, 1982) criticized the central delivery suite provision for maternity services. The report maintained that 'Nucleus' incorporated a higher patient turnover rate than could be realized in normal practice. Such studies highlighted a hidden pressure within 'Nucleus' to change the nature of hospital work organization. Within the tighter space planning of the 'Nucleus' departments the only means of maintaining output was to make more intensive use of facilities by such measures as longer shifts and the use of spaces for several purposes. To achieve equivalent output in a smaller hospital implies the modification of informal systems of bed control employed by consultants and the elimination of such practices as deliberate 'bed blocking'.

The inability of hospital administrators to achieve such changes meant that patient throughput was unlikely to increase with 'Nucleus'. Indeed in the case reported by Vann-Wye (1986) the intention to preserve current work practices was present at the planning stage. In this case the Central Treatment Area facilities were actually eliminated. Whilst this move was argued in terms of revenue costs it meant that surgery in shifts was ruled out. Day surgery was opposed by medical staff within the Area Health Authority. This case provides a detailed illustration of how the liberaliz-ation of 'Nucleus' design policies was brought about. Pressure for change was applied by lower tier authorities upon the department. During this process of design adaptation key influence was exerted by medical and nursing professionals who aimed at higher space standards. In certain parts of the Newtown design (see Chapter 13), the space allocations of 'Nucleus' were seriously breached and the final hospital design represented a sub-stantial increase upon 'Nucleus' limits. Such events in individual hospital project deliberations can be taken to explain the changes in departmental stance voiced by a DHSS office in October 1982 (Vann-Wye, 1986).

> When first developed it was anticipated that users would simply take the published Data Pack material and work through it to tender documents, thence to construction stages. The Data Packs were put together with the fairly certain knowledge that some trimming would need to be done to suit particular circumstances in individual hospitals. As things have turned out the use of the 'Nucleus' material has been much wider than any of us envisaged initially. At one end of the scale the 'Nucleus' policies have been abstracted from the Data Packs and themselves used to generate new designs. Between these limits we have seen all manner of combinations and permutations.

Competing ideologies of care

The dominance of the hospital sector within the NHS and its importance in private medical care derives from the interplay of different ideologies of health care. Hospital treatment for the wealthy did not become fashionable until the last quarter of the 19th century. This is understandable, given the antecedents of the hospitals as an institutional type. A private fee-paying clientele was unlikely to be attracted by a treatment environment deriving from the barrack room and the poor-house. Not until the medical profession organized with a coherent system of ethics and training, and not until rival professional groups had been subjugated (see Chapter 1) were hospitals seen for what they could be: large and prestigious units whose work was underpinned by a rationale of scientific medicine.

Before the growth of the hospital system, the model for private medicine had been treatment of the patient at home. This kind of care may be labelled 'individualistic-curative' and was entrepreneurial in character. The sanitary reforms of the 19th century produced striking improvements in mobility and mortality statistics. Measures such as the construction of sewers and the provision of clean water had dramatic effects upon the control of contagion. These works were 'communal-preventative' in character and municipally funded.

The former approach offered a career structure for gifted and socially well-connected doctors. By way of contrast the latter method of tackling disease relied heavily upon basic hygiene and infrastructural sanitary provision. Its effects were generalized and anonymous. These two philosophies of health care – 'cure' and 'prevention' – represented distinct methods of attacking problems of morbidity. In the UK the former became associated with private practice and the latter with local authority and state finance.

The advent of a state-funded service in 1947 posed a choice. There was a possibility of giving primacy to a curative, practitioner-centred service or a communal programme of preventative health care. With the granting of clinical freedom to the medical profession, the curative model gained dominance through state sponsorship of the hospital service. The status accorded to hospital consultants as leaders of developments in specialist treatment led to the promotion of a highly capitalized hospital service which took precedence over the community-based general practitioner.

The elevation of hospital-based care over other treatment techniques was aided by other factors. Building new hospitals was a tangible way of demonstrating political achievement. In a climate of post-War reconstruction it was a vote-winner. Wartime rationing may have had positive virtues in promoting a good, if sparse, diet, but self-denial soon lost its appeal in the consumer boom of the late 1950s and early 1960s. Government was expected 'to deliver the goods' and new hospitals formed part of that package. Hospitals were to become the most capital-and-revenue-intensive part of the service. Within their walls, technologically-based treatments could be researched and implemented out of the public purse. These techniques could then be readily used by NHS consultants on a fee-for-service basis in the private sector.

It has been shown how the assembly of a district design database for public hospitals was delayed until the 1960s. Shortages in post-War development funds had led to the extension and adaptation of existing premises. By the time expansion could be contemplated, departmental and regional designers had already become accustomed to a policy of incremental modification. Suggestions for radical change in policy approaches encountered a situation in which the dominant curative mode was being preserved by the maintenance of the existing building stock. The inheritance of established hospitals provided strong models for layout and work organization.

In principle the questions posed for NHS hospital designers were several, whether or not they were perceived in their full sharpness:

- What kinds of facilities should be provided?
- Should the NHS hospital take its model from private practice and feature single-room accommodation with hotel-type services?
- Should traditional open-ward forms be preserved?
- Was the hospital to be conceived as a hostel providing bed and board within a community-centred environment?
- Was the model of industrial organization to be adopted with an emphasis placed upon capital intensive central treatment areas and operating facilities?
- What role should hospitals play in preventative health care programmes – had they a role in health education?
- What was a hospital's proper relationship to the community it served, and what should this involve in terms of out-patient and clinic work?

These were some of the more general design policy issues. Other areas which required definition concerned architectural and hence corporate imagery. Hospitals had long functioned as foci for community self-identification. They were symbols of prestige and acted as civic monuments within urban landscapes. Should designers strive for monolithic images of institutional power or should the NHS project the façade of routine factory production? Should hospitals be unique and striking in their external appearance or should they look like the uniform appendages of a nationwide system of service outlets?

There were several routes to resolving this complex of criteria (Calderhead, 1975; Stone, 1980). In terms of visual appearance it is difficult to isolate general tendencies other than saying that on the whole, buildings were modest in scale and adopted a highly articulated plan-form. In the years of 'one-off' designing when Regional Health Authorities used private firms of designers individual differences in appearance remained quite marked. Common tendencies tended to derive from DHSS recommendations on space limits and departmental layouts. What does seem to have emerged from early essays in hospital design was a conventional wisdom about how the general pattern of departmental relationships should be shaped. This knowledge of departmental relationships and overall patterns of configuration for hospitals seems to have become part of the design folklore of the service.

This constituted a hidden table of criticality in which the degree of centrality of each department to the work flow was assessed. An informal ranking arose which gave each department a weighting in the competition for prime territorial position. Such shared assumptions became embedded in DHSS and regional 'operational policies', which were the mode of specifying work flow relationships within projected developments. Those specializations involved in acute care or in crucial diagnostic procedures tended to gain prime locations. For example, operating theatres and X-ray departments score highly in departmental territorial rankings. Their association with high levels of engineering services and expensive capital equipment buttresses their status. Thus the priority of acute medical specialisms is built into the NHS planning culture. The previously mentioned case study showed that extra resources which become available during a hospital planning cycle will tend to be appropriated by acute medical and surgical specialisms. The same study also demonstrated that times of financial crisis in individual hospital developments lead to a diversion of funds from geriatric services to acute care specialisms despite government policies to the contrary. Thus the priority tagging of certain specialisms creates a drift towards the enhancement of provision for acute specialisms at the expense of specialisms such as mental health and geriatrics, whose palliative treatment regimes are regarded as less crucial.

Paradoxically 'Best Buy' was represented as a cheap whole hospital design which was avowedly part of a policy of increasing emphasis upon community-based care. Early discharge was to remove the convalescent function from hospitals but in doing so it intensified their role as providers of therapy for acute conditions. The use of Central Treatment Areas in 'Best Buy' designs was part of this intensification philosophy. The production of the 'Harness' design material marked an increase in the scale of acute hospital facilities. The 'Harness' format represented the high-water mark in the provision of a technologically intensive NHS plant.

'Nucleus' returned to a far more domestic scale. Being only a planning system, it left regional designers discretion in the choice of building, construction and finishes. However, the recommended constructional methods and building techniques were widely promulgated by the DHSS. However, the designers retained the philosophy of early patient discharge. The 'Nucleus' ward layout with its nurses' station positioned in the centre of the half-cruciform layout presumed a patient population of high dependency cases.

Competing technologies of care

Given the underlying curative bias evident in the NHS health care methodologies, it may seem strange to speak of 'competing' technologies of care. Yet 'care' is not divisible into specific areas of competence related to the exclusive treatment of individual pathologies. Medicine is not an unambiguous science. There are alternative treatments for any given condition. Thus medical and paramedical specialisms are in competition for patients and for the facilities with which to treat them. As we have described in previous chapters the system of competitive bidding for resources in the hospital design process represents a contest for resources between professional specialisms. This means that within each development project the final hospital content and forms of work organization cannot be precisely preconceptualized at the early planning stages. Given the power of professions to determine the physical and socio-technical details of design, the main thrust of NHS design practice has been to regard buildings as shells for equipment rather than as working organizations housing people. The significance of intra-organizational resource contests within a decentralized design system has meant that spatial and territorial considerations become dominant over attempts to re-shape systematically the work flows within the hospital shell.

The effect of this political geometry of design can be said to have affected the nature of the knowledge bases developed by the DHSS. These have generally sought to impose space and cost limits rather than to approach the fine detail of work organization. 'DHSS Building Notes, Technical Memoranda', and the system of Cost Allowances can all be seen in this light. Similarly the departmental 'Capricode' system used to process regional project submissions has examination of physical provisions as its chief aim. 'Capricode' is used by the central department as a delay mechanism in addition to its monitoring of standards. This system of delay was issued to meet the overall needs of the Treasury Department (Turner, 1970, 1971; Vann-Wye 1986). Whilst DHSS officers can use 'Capricode' to promote delay by the elaboration of technical criticisms, they can do little to stipulate the final patterns of clinical practice which new hospitals will house.

A second source of constraint might be discovered in 'rationalized' construction methods. The use of prefabrication in some of the wartime emergency provision furnished an example of what could be done, but not until the early 1960s did government espouse industrialized building methods. The practice of 'one-off' designing then present in hospital architecture militated against the achievement of large savings and the establishment of standard constructional techniques. Some public sector enterprises such as education took up rationalized construction methods, notably in the design of schools in Hertfordshire. The appointment of Tatton Brown as first Ministry Chief Architect led to a steering of design in a systems direction. The promotion of departmental databases provided a common core of practice around which building approaches could develop upon a coordinated modular basis. Some regions, notably Oxford Regional Health Authority, took up this system building potential and evolved constructional methods of their own.

Yet it would be a mistake to overplay the role of industrialized building in hospital design. Industrialized techniques rapidly ran into problems throughout the public sector. These were often caused by the misuse of materials in design or in actual construction and lack of hierarchical discipline in the process of building. But each system employed different mixes of raw materials. With changing prices and periodic shortages of certain materials, the relative cost advantages of different methods could change quickly. Considered alongside the relatively long development periods of hospital projects, this phenomenon could mean that cost savings could be lost by the time a scheme came to the construction stage. Likewise, the policy of phasing developments over several years compromised system building advantages. The outcome of the process has thus left hospital design in an ambivalent relationship *vis-à-vis* rationalized building methods. The promulgated standards generally eschewed attachment to a service-wide system of prefabricated construction. The most successful exemplar, 'Nucleus', was a rationalized planning system which left constructional methods to Regional Health Authority discretion. Its cost-saving advantages were to be gained from providing a limited vocabulary of layouts to which building contractors could become accustomed.

A third configuration of constraints emerged with the growth of the state-directed medical provision, as the major client of the medical supplies industry. Instead of confronting a large number of individual hospitals under different kinds of control, equipment and pharmaceutical manufacturers could develop products to meet a more homogeneous clientele. Liaison between the NHS and manufacturers became part of the design process. An examination of technical information sheets produced for standard designs like those of the DHSS demonstrates the closeness of this relationship between user and supplier.

The 'Nucleus' project in particular revealed the degree of multi-dimensional coordination needed between equipment makers and the central design agency. By setting down recommended space and planning standards, the assembly of organized configurations of plant and equipment enabled hospital planning to take place within routine and rule-bound procedures. This process opened up the possibility of marketing design packages. The DHSS saw in its work the opportunity for the export of design. This trend reached a climax with the 'Nucleus' design material where marketing efforts have taken place at an international level in combination with equipment suppliers. This transfer of technology was facilitated by the considerable influence of UK medical training abroad.

By the 1980s, the movement into 'community care' also provided a spur to the design of long-term palliative care for groups such as the elderly within the private sector. These private nursing homes often depend upon NHS facilities for expensive equipment or sophisticated laboratory services. Thus the existence of a complementarity between private and public provision, with the modes of the former heavily dependent on the latter, can be seen to have emerged over the last decade.

Yet notwithstanding the variations evidenced in working hospitals, one can discern general template configurations in the way that hospitals are conceived. There is considerable agreement about what a hospital of a particular type should be like. This knowledge derives from operating experience and constitutes a generalized recipe for devising layouts. The most significant design effort is expended upon departmental configurations. Hospital planning is viewed as a linking together of separate departments by circulation areas. Initial consideration tends to be given to departmental functioning across and within a communications network with engineering services provision being tailored to this. Estimates of traffic flow and tests of adequacy for circulation spaces are made at individual project level. They often use the estimated number of journeys between departmental areas derived from customary practice. Such measures do not affect the total conception of work design in a way which seeks to re-shape jobs to reduce movement.

Indeed the continuation of design templates rests fundamentally on the exercise of a global form of institutionalized power expressed in various micro-circuits of local influence. In the case studied by Vann-Wye (1986) the decisive influence of district and regional medical and nursing staff upon final hospital layout is clearly present. In these inter-occupational negotiations, standard design materials become benchmarks used to push for increased resource. The project architects tended to act as 'honest brokers', compromising rival claims or acting as mere technicians drawing up the provisions stipulated by medical and other groups. Extra-organizational interests in the guise of the local New Town Development Corporation acted to preserve the project when medical staff in existing district hospitals finally opposed it.

Therefore at the level of individual project design the influence of regional and district medical staff tends to be crucial. Practitioners in existing district units often take a strong role in determining the scope and content of each new hospital. Their own particular patterns of practice will tend to be designed into the new unit. Thus the layout of NHS hospitals is usually shaped by inter- and intra-professional contests for resources. The ability of each individual to secure space and place is conditioned by a range of factors including:

- His/her social skills and organizational political connections within and beyond the local health authority concerned.
- The status ranking of his/her occupation within the NHS; and within each discipline the generally perceived centrality of his/her activity within the work flow of health care provision.

Without doubt DHSS influence in hospitals has been consolidated since the establishment of the NHS. There now exists an extensive database to guide regional designers and to police their proposals. However, the advent of standardized design material has not brought about departmental hegemony in design expertise. Much adaptation and discretion is still exercised at Regional Health Authority level. The likelihood of the acceptance of departmental design information has increased with the imposition of other kinds of budgetary restrictions upon lower tier authorities.

Backing into the future

Taking a long-term perspective it may be said that (former) DHSS standard exemplar designs have exerted their strongest influence when they have been combined with measures of financial restraint. The widespread influence of 'Nucleus' can be traced to service-wide funding reductions. Given tight budgets, regions were compelled to give recognition to 'Nucleus' design templates. Adoption of 'Nucleus' principles meant the possibility of continuing hospital construction. Penalties of not adopting the standard materials were higher design costs, longer approvals procedures and the probability of losing projects altogether.

What the 1974 cases did was to destroy the image of the NHS as the provider of comprehensive 'state-of-the-art' health care. With 'Nucleus' came a cheaper and shoddier level of provision, more intensive usage of premises, earlier discharge policies and a greater reliance upon the community services. 'Nucleus', with its initial £6 m price tag represented a retreat from ever more ambitious projections of hospital-based health care provision service. It was recommended not only for new whole hospital developments but in a 'tack-on' role to existing buildings. It could therefore be viewed as compatible with a return to 'make do and mend' policies. An important stipulation in the 'Nucleus' design philosophy was the idea of new 'Nucleus' hospitals being dependent upon existing units for support services. This designed dependency attempted to forestall the establishment of large functionally independent units.

Apart from these fundamental re-orientations in design policy, financial difficulties began to beset individual hospital development schemes. These problems became especially pressing during the early 1980s when the Conservative Government sought to impose restrictions upon the number of projects advanced for development by RHAs. The 'Rayner Letter' sent by the DHSS to RHAs in late 1982 caused a re-ordering of building priorities throughout the service. As time went on and the Government's expenditure restrictions bit deeper, hospital building programmes became subject to unpredictable delays and postponements. Long-term planning projections were seriously compromised.

This tradition of piecemeal re-design of hospitals can be seen to have seriously impeded the introduction of information technology (IT) particularly in the form of 'smart buildings'. Although hospital planners may talk much about the implications of IT for the working of new hospital units, little has been done to anticipate these elements in designing new units or incorporating them in the pre-commissioning stages. The actual selection and 'plumbing in' of the systems to be used tends to be left to the commissioning and post-commissioning stages. Similarly in the design of hospitals the opportunities for CAD have not been realized to the full. The retreat from 'Harness' meant an abandonment of computer-based methods. Employment of a computer-aided methodology by the (former) DHSS and its application to standard designs could undoubtedly reduce design periods. That such steps have not been taken is probably due to the autonomy granted to Regions and Districts in detailed design matters. There is little point in the central department designing at a rapid speed if time is frittered away by extensive modifications by lower tier authorities. Effective introduction of CAD techniques thus waits upon a re-design of the NHS planning and design system as a whole.

In principle, it would be possible to design the physical shell and work organization together. Given a reasonably short timescale in commissioning it would be possible to realize this pre-conceptualized entity in new buildings housing the pre-planned working arrangements. However, within the present NHS procedures for the design of work and workplace these processes seldom take place simultaneously. The planning and design of a new hospital work organization is only conceived in terms of a generalized system of intra- and inter-departmental activity flows taking place within the physical envelope. This is not only because of changing circumstances and a prolonged design period precludes detailed planning at an early stage, but was also because the line managers, that is the consultants who are to hold operational responsibility are not consulted until the commissioning or immediate post-commissioning stages. For this reason structural modifications can begin soon after the new hospital has opened!

Commissioning a new hospital is a relatively uncommon experience for personnel. Commissioning literature is relatively sparse and unorganized. The general NHS experience has been one of commissioning additions to existing premises. Here the insertion of a new development into an already established institution has to recognize the existing range of practices and power structures. It could be said that this adaptive method of re-design has been carried into the commissioning of new units built on green field sites. There is little conscious re-thinking of the form of work organization design intentions incorporated in the physical shell.

However, there is a medical hegemony which is exerted over the size and organization of hospital spaces in a diversity of ways from the most diffuse to the highly specific. Most of the fine texture of work designing occurs through the colonization of buildings by staffs with strong shared expectations of the nature of work organization and culture. Such professional constraints on hospital design have meant that changes in hospital form and operation tend to be slow. The response of the system to sudden changes in extra-organizational conditions is limited. The changed behavioural circumstances implied by macro-economic constraints can be difficult to implement with any speed and certainty. The negotiated nature of policy changes, mediated through complex administrative structures has enabled established ideologies to define the nature of innovation in plant and equipment.

Modes of central and regional resource allocation have failed to erode established inequalities. Mechanisms such as the Regional Allocation White Paper (RAWP) formulae sought a redistribution of resources, but inequalities remain that are difficult to eradicate. These inequalities are preserved in many ways, not least amongst which is the loyalty with which local hospitals are supported by their local communities. Health authorities often experience difficulties in closing units or in re-distributing facilities due to local community opposition. District Health Authorities may thus not be able to apportion limited resources in the light of strict economic criteria.

Placing such considerations aside, it must be said that a crucial weakness of welfare economic criteria has been that internal NHS contests for resources waste money in terms of the time taken to reach agreed allocations. There is much 'overdesign' of hospitals to local requirements. Often such design outputs are chronically obsolescent by the time they are realized in built form. Furthermore, professional competition for capital and for the territorial segregation of departments can have resulted in unnecessary duplication of facilities. It is against this background that the proposed new legislation on hospital management must be approached. As has been suggested in previous chapters the new measures are designed to promote the process of rationalization initiated by Florence Nightingale. They are based on the same concept of individual curative principles that has driven the professional contest for resources in the emergent forms of 'industrialized' health care provision. Indeed the present Government may be seen to be seeking to force this contest into the marketplace where it can be better articulated through consumer devices. A necessary complement to this process might be seen to be a greatly extended emphasis on the collective prevention of ill health rather than upon individualistic curative modes and a massive re-direction of resources to this end.

References

Abel-Smith, B. (1964) *The Hospital 1800–1948*. London: Heinemann.
Alexander, C. (1979) *The Timeless Way of Building*. New York: Oxford University Press.
Bevan, A. (1976) *In Place of Fear*. Wakefield: E.P. Publishing.
Bonham Carter, Sir A. (1969) *The Functions of the District General Hospital (Bonham Carter Report)*. London: DHSS.
British Medical Association News Review (1976) Nucleus hospitals: a springboard or a trap? *BMANR*, **1**(13), May, 205–6.
British Medical Journal (1976) Nucleus hospitals. *BMJ*, **1**(6004), 31 January, 245–6.
Calderhead, J. (1975) *Hospitals for People: A Look at Some New Buildings in England*. London: King Edward's Hospital Fund.
Central Health Services Council (1969) *The Function of the District General Hospital*. London: HMSO.
Checkletts, J. *et al.* (1982) *Split in the nucleus. Health and Social Service Journal*, **XCII** (4792), 15 April, 473–6.
DHSS/COI (1973) *Best Buy Hospitals*. London: HMSO.
DHSS (1976) *Nucleus*. London: DHSS.

DHSS (1982) *Reports 1–6, Steering Group of Health Service Information* (Chair: Mrs E. Körner).
Foot, M. (1973) *Aneurin Bevan: A Biography. Vol. 2. 1945–1960.* London: Davis-Poynter.
Forty, A. (1980) The modern hospital in England and France: The social and medical uses of architecture. In: King, A.D. (ed.) *Buildings and Society: Essays on Social Development of the Built Environment,* pp. 61–93. London: Routledge and Kegan Paul.
Foucault, M. (1977) *Discipline and Punish: The Birth of the Prison.* London: Allen Lane.
Gainsborough, H. and Gainsborough, J. (1964) *Principles of Hospital Design.* London: The Architectural Press.
Green, J. (1971) *Hospital Research and Briefing Problems.* London: King Edward's Hospital Fund.
Griffiths, R. (1983) *NHS Management Enquiry Document,* 6th October.
Health and Social Services Journal (1979) A phoenix from the ashes. *HSSJ,* **LXXXIX** (4635), 30 March, 336–7.
HMSO (1976) *Priorities in Health and Personal Social Services in England.* London: HMSO.
Holroyd, W.A.H. (ed.) (1968) *Hospital Traffic and Supply Problems.* London: King Edward's Hospital Fund.
James, P. (1974) Critical comment on Harness. *Health and Social Services Journal,* **LXXXIV**(4393), 29 June, 1441.
King Edward's Hospital Fund (1981) *The Planning and Organization of Nucleus Hospitals,* K.F.C. 81/17. London: King's Fund Centre.
Kuhn, T.S. (1962) *The Structure of Scientific Revolutions.* Chicago: University of Chicago Press.
McFarlane, J. *et al.* (1980) *Hospitals in the NHS,* Project Paper 15. London: King's Fund Centre.
Merton, R.K. (1973) *The Sociology of Science: Theoretical and Empirical Investigations.* Chicago: University of Chicago Press.
MESS (1982) *Biochemistry Laboratory No. 1 – A Case Study Report* (1st Draft). Birmingham: Faculty of Management and Policy Sciences, University of Aston.
MESS (1985) *New Technologies in Banking, Retailing and Health Services.* Birmingham: ESRC Work Organization Research Centre, University of Aston.
Ministry of Health (1962) *A Hospital Plan for England and Wales.* London: HMSO.
Ministry of Health (1966) *The Hospital Building Programme: A Revision of the Hospital Plan For England and Wales.* London: HMSO.
Nightingale, F. (1864) *Notes on Hospitals.* London: Longman, Green Longman, Roberts and Green.
Noakes, A. (1982) DHSS development projects: An architectural history. *Health Services Estate,* No. 48, April, 118–30.
Nuffield Provincial Hospitals Trust (1955) *Studies in the Functions and Design of Hospitals.* London: Oxford University Press.
O'Neill, B. (1980) Harness hospitals die in mid-operation. *New Civil Engineer,* No. 396, 5 June, 36–7.
RIBA (1960) *Trends in Planning: RIBA Hospitals Course Handbook. Papers given at the Royal Institute of British Architects.* London: RIBA Technical Information Services.

Schutz, A. (1972) *The Phenomenology of the Social World*. London: Heinemann.

Stone, P. (ed.) (1980) *British Hospital and Health Care Buildings: Designs and Appraisals*. London: Architectural Press.

Turner, B.A. (1970) *The Cost Effectiveness of Hospital Design: Fieldwork Feedback Report*, June. Departments of Civil Engineering and Social Sciences and Economics, University of Loughborough.

Turner, B.A. (1971) *Research in Cost Control Procedures in Hospital Construction for the Department of Health and Social Security: Briefing Procedures*, March. Departments of Civil Engineering and Social Sciences and Economics, University of Loughborough.

Vann-Wye, G.M. (1986) Designing Technical Change: A Study within the National Health Service, PhD Thesis. Birmingham: University of Aston.

Welsh Office (1979) *Use of Nucleus Design Material*, HBSS 130/141/1, January. Cardiff: Welsh Office.

Wilkinson, B. (1983) *The Shopfloor Politics of New Technology*. London: Heinemann.

13 | Reconstructing the Future: The Politics of Designing a New Hospital

Sudi Sharifi

This chapter discusses the activities of a set of health planners and administrators in a District Health Authority (DHA), 'Bordershire', who were involved in the planning, design and commissioning of a District General Hospital (DGH). The DGH was designed to provide health service for some 250 000 inhabitants of a new town and its surrounding areas in England. It was planned and designed according to 'Nucleus' principles instigated by a government department (the then DHSS). The 'Nucleus' building system was chosen by the department to accelerate the process of design and commissioning of the DGH and to reduce the time and cost elements in the DHA's capital programme. The chapter includes analysis and interpretation of the events which provided the grounds for the administrators' planning decisions and other activities. It is divided into two parts. Part I provides an overview of the observed and reported events, negotiations between the involved agencies as regards the planning and commissioning of the DGH. Part II includes an interpretation and analysis of these events and negotiations. It outlines the intended actions of these actors in transforming the established planning practices and procedures and reconstructing some of the key events within their identified contexts.

I Negotiating design

In providing a case for building a new hospital at 'Newtown' DHA officers from 'Bordershire District' at first highlighted the deficiency of local services and the socio-economic deprivation of the area. The DHA as the user was later required to negotiate with the Regional Health Authority (RHA) officers and DHSS on the type of building design suitable for Newtown. The 'Nucleus' design system was recommended by the government department to the RHA's Project Team as the most suitable building system for the new DGH. There were two stages in the approval of the final design. In the initial stage the principles and criteria on which the design was based were discussed. This was followed by considerations of the details and required modifications and adjustments. The issues were discussed in meetings of the Project Team involving both planners and administrators from the Regional District. The Region's architects interpreted the 'Nucleus' principles for the participants.

Whilst providing a basic core of DGH patient services, the 'Nucleus' system was expected to make maximum use of existing facilities and services. The officers assumed that adopting the 'Nucleus' design standard did not imply conforming in a prescribed fashion. Consequently, 'Nucleus' was defined as a 'beginning' in the decision-making process. Necessary modifications could be added later if it fell short of the DHA requirements. Members of the planning team in Bordershire DHA, therefore, claimed that they actually challenged the principles of the 'Nucleus' design as laid down by the DHSS. Such a challenge could not have been easy, since any modification to the standardized design required DHSS approval before it was incorporated into the system. This government department had the powers to reject any proposed modifications or to disregard the timetables through delaying approval. The modified pieces of design had first to be approved by both the RHA and the project team before being implemented. The RHA officers owned the technical know-how on the design's merits. Yet, the DHA planners and administrators were in the position of defining local needs and the type and standard of required services.

At the time when planning for the DGH started, the 'Nucleus' design package was at its early stages of establishment yet it was presented in a form that could be taken up and amplified by any design team. The planners in the DHA said that they 'copied all the details' of the standard 'Nucleus' pack. Contrarily, they claimed that they had departed from the standard design whilst considering the positioning of some of the departments within the layout, for example Central Treatment Areas (CTAs). The CTA was defined as a unit where the nurses took the patients off the ward for treatment. This was a provision for all patients. The actors at the time considered the environment for altering the concept of CTA as 'top notch', i.e. they could put their 're-invention' into practice. The nurse planner involved articulated this argument based upon both technical and professional understandings. The role was seen as that of 'positioning' the CTA within the prescribed layout according to various aspects of nurse training. The final positioning of the CTA would restrain the nurse's monitoring of patients' progress and of the nurse's responses also.

As a 'clinical specialist', a sister was expected to have a clear idea of the nature of the physical treatments available. In a CTA he or she would not always be working on a particular area of speciality so would have to rely on the information given second hand. The CTA would generate traffic problems in the continuous movement of beds and nurses from wards to the treatment area. Furthermore, in the DHSS's design blueprint the CTA was located on the ground floor which meant the patients in wards on the first floor would have to be taken down by the lifts or other means. These problems led to a modification of the 'Nucleus' design template. In order to overcome the training and traffic difficulties the planners in Bordershire DHA thought of designing 'local treatment areas'. They negotiated their modifications through the members of the project team at the RHA in order to obtain the approval of the DHSS. They used the technical expertise of the Regional Officers because, they argued, this would gain them credibility and allies in bargaining nationally.

In fact they were successful in their appeal and afterwards claimed that the variations that they introduced into the CTA were thereafter included in the 'Nucleus Pack'. It was known that such changes in the basic design concepts originating with DHAs were rare. Nevertheless, in the process of commissioning of Newtown DGH the officers increasingly seemed to treat the 'Nucleus' planning system as an end in itself and the 'Nucleus' concept became the frame of reference for service planning and fundings, despite its limitations.

Planning for a hospital and the recommended team approach

The concept of 'District General Hospital' (DGH) originated in the 1962 Hospital Plan. It was described as a large, complex hospital which served a large population and required a complex management organization. The concept became popular mainly because of the 1960s' social forces. In that era there was an 'engineering approach' to medicine which considered human beings as complex machines. The DGH was thus considered as the 'health factory' because it contained high medical technology. According to the DHA officers in Bordershire this system also served to meet the status needs of the medical profession. It also served the interests of the state as fund-providers in rationalizing the financial and logistical planning of the NHS and in increasing the efficiency of the non-medical services.

The early 1980s restructuring of the NHS made the DHA become the 'basic' planning unit. Planning decisions were to be devolved to the local level and 'left to local discretion'. Two main components of the planning system remained untouched: (1) 'strategic' plans would still be prepared by Local (now District) and Regional Officers every five years, taking into account 10-year prospects in health service; and (2) the 'annual programme of action' which was to be prepared for two years in advance by the Local (District) administrators alongside their strategic plans. The DHSS put forward a set of principles which were expected to make the planning efforts of the District Officers more effective. Emphasis was put on a consultative and collaborative planning process; more particularly on the involvement of various staff and professional groups. Thereafter planning became a 'part of the management function', a continuous process rather than a series of *ad hoc* events.

Newtown DGH was the most major project considered in Bordershire's strategic plan for the 1980s. Improvement of the standard of existing health provisions was the object of this strategic plan. The adopted processes of decision making attempted to reproduce the DHSS planning guidelines. The Newtown Hospital project was carried through by a set of teams: a design team, a project team and a manpower and commissioning team. According to the manuals on procedures for building a hospital, teams were significant elements in the hospital development process. The manuals were themselves produced by various research institutions for health planning, and contained detailed guidelines on the structure of these teams, their membership and how their activities should be organized.

The project team (PT) was therefore to be composed of representatives of the different professions involved in hospital design, building and hospital administration, nursing and medical activities. The PT meetings had to be held monthly. The items on their agenda required the representation of Newtown Development Corporation in order to negotiate certain commitments and of some medical consultants to provide the 'team' with expert advice on particular design questions, e.g. hospital traffic. The DHA was represented by the nurse planner and general administrator (planning) in these meetings. The PT worked on the broad assumption that Newtown DGH was *one* of the hospital building projects which was being organized nationally at the time. Hence when they decided on the scope of its services according to the 'Nucleus' standards they assumed that these were being followed by others and that matters such as number of wards, operating theatres and their location, etc. would accord with national standards. Yet these decisions were submitted to detailed and prolonged discussions, involving the professionals on the PT. They assumed that the DHA acted as a 'semi-autonomous body' whilst handling the corporate strategies of the DHSS. The members of the District Management Team (DMT) thus might be seen to have assumed that their role was the implementation of 'strategic plans' through a rearrangement of the national elements. Similarly, the second-in-line officers, mainly members of the Manpower and Commissioning Team (MCT) for Newtown DGH, developed a set of interpretive frameworks designed to implement these guidelines.

At first the DMT had set their strategies with reference to the DHSS objectives of several years before in 1978. These strategies were extensions of patterns developed prior to the reorganization of the NHS in 1974. The adoption of a resource spreading policy by the NHS in the 1960s had led to 'deliberate' ministerial action which emphasized the needs of 'Cinderella' services, i.e. geriatric and psychiatric services. This slowly evolved logic set the design parameters for a 'Nucleus' hospital prototype.

However, at local level the DHA's customary approach, as regards hospital building, had been to plan for the local need for services as defined by local professionals and then apply for the capital from the RHA. This approach occasionally brought frustration in the late 1970s, as resources became constrained nationally and the local managers were faced with logistical problems. The members of the Bordershire MCT argued that in a system like the NHS the 'identification of the markets for their services' was central to its operations. However, the national DHSS guidelines for the 1970s had provided a different direction in this context for the DHA members of the PT. The functional content of Newtown DGH was planned in relation to the historical priority attached to Cinderella services. The most recent re-structuring of the NHS management system seemed to have little effect on the planning priorities of the DHA officers in the DMT over the period of the 1980s. This was illustrated in their 'confidence in the continuity' of Newtown DGH project. In other words the 'routine work' of the DHA was seen as remaining unchanged by distant signals such as the Griffiths Report and talk of 'rationalization'.

Activities of the Manpower and Commissioning Team (MCT)

The MCT was established in order to finalize the design details and examine the structural options for the hospital and its manpower. In the early stages of its establishment the members of the MCT arranged their meetings on a monthly basis and organized their activities accordingly. Over a period of two years as the financial policy of the Health Authority changed and delays were imposed on the opening date of the DGH, the frequency of the meetings of the MCT decreased. The team comprised of the second-in-line officers in the DHA who had worked within the NHS system for a long time. Some of them were qualified nurses who climbed the managerial ladder in the District and Regional Health Authorities in different parts of the UK. Some of the younger members joined the NHS with management and planning experiences which they had acquired in private and commercial organizations. The DMT officers took part in the MCT meetings and provided information, advice and reassurance with regard to the items on the agenda. The involvement of the medical consultants decreased as delays on the building projects were imposed.

At its inauguration meeting, the MCT developed a 'working plan'. The assumed tasks were to be executed through 'sub-groups', to each of which at least one member of the PT was attached as convenor. The sub-groups developed 'task lists' on an annual basis. The items on the agenda of the MCT meetings circulated around the activities of these sub-groups in turn. There were time deadlines set by the MCT and PT for various tasks of the sub-groups in order to ensure the progress of the project. The sub-groups also worked as task forces providing the technical/specialist know-how required by the MCT to fulfil its objectives. They reported back to the MCT monthly. On the basis of these reports the MCT submitted bi-annual reports to the DMT.

The MCT members argued that since the building of the Newtown Hospital would be accompanied by the 'rationalization' of services within the District and the need to recruit new staff for the DGH, public relations activities should be an essential part of the commissioning process. They were encouraged to take 'every opportunity to speak to local community groups about the hospital' and to familiarize the local inhabitants with the likely organization of the new hospital. The most uncertain, yet controlling, issue for the MCT was the continuance and the availability of funding for the Newtown DGH Project. In the same period the DHSS started planning for 'efficiency cuts' which implied financial squeezes on the health authorities' budgets, in particular on their development projects. The revenue consequences of the DGH approval implied the closure of at least ten of the old cottage hospitals in the surrounding area as well as numerous wards in other hospitals. Hence the commissioning of Newtown DGH was a major exercise for the whole of Bordershire DHA. It involved a large number of present and potential actors and initiated considerable changes in the organization and distribution of health services in the district.

The selection of hospitals for closure was largely a 'political process' as the DHA correspondence with other bodies showed it involved the interference of local MPs during election campaigns throughout the 1980s and required extensive negotiation with various interest groups. During the course of commissioning, the primary forecasts of resources were revised several times as the funding circumstances changed and efficiency savings imposed on the design of the hospital. The officers had constantly to re-draw a balance between capital expenditure and revenue consequences of the DGH. Although the MCT established a finance and approval sub-group, the financial appraisal activities were not actually integrated into the commissioning process. The MCT became involved in financial debates however, because of the General Administrator's membership of the Resource Allocation Working Party (RAWP).

II The commissioning process: an interpretation and analysis

Meetings and roles-sets

The process of commissioning Newtown DGH involved long-term negotiations and discussions over the underlying assumptions of the Nucleus Planning System, interpretation of these assumptions and selection of approaches to various problems. The MCT for Newtown DGH acted like a clearing house for these tasks and for mediating different approaches. In their meetings usually everyone reported on the outcomes of their 'persuasive' activities and their attempts in 'selling the DGH' to medical consultants and the sub-group convenors reported on their activities. Certain issues and points raised by members were noted by the chairman which sometimes led to the re-setting of assignments or tasks which were to be undertaken by the members. The members of the team used their regular monthly meetings to develop and maintain a united front with respect to proposed developments and revenue implications. The meetings were for the major actors who informed others of the latest changes and the news about the approvals or refusals. They provided the opportunity for the officers:

- to clarify their stance against the members of other groups,
- to decide on their 'philosophies' and 'strategies' as regards the DGH project, and
- to identify tactics for handling interest groups.

The debates in the MCT meetings elaborated the gaps in the members' preferred approaches to manpower issues. Some actors gave priority to the reaction of the 'biggies', i.e. the Heads of Departments in the existing District hospital. This was because if the DHA showed any interest in the future recruitment of their existing staff, they wanted to intervene to ask, 'what's in it for us?' Members of the MCT attempted to agree on the way they could 'win over' current medical staff when they wanted them to join the project. The recruitment of key medical staff dominated the MCT debates on future staffing. The aim was to get them to sign a DHA contract in order to make the situation more controllable. Hence, 'lobbying' them, 'selling the "Nucleus" idea' and 'introducing the DGH as an entity' were the recipes 'to stop the fight'. Paradoxically, as their efforts to co-opt key personnel grew more intense, these second-in-line administrative officers assumed roles in opposition to the medical staff. The latter became identified as the most powerful group in the situation and one which could pose a threat to the momentum of the commissioning process. These issues were frequently raised in the MCT meetings and were often used by the planners as a latent sanction to modify the members' positions.

One of the major issues extensively discussed in these meetings was the possible delays in the DHSS or RHA approval of the main building contract. Related events were noted and the outcomes of the events were speculated upon, but this did not imply that substantive decision might follow. The MCT operated as a working group and had no authority to function as a decision-making body. The actors examined various ways that tasks allocated to sub-groups could be handled and consensually selected 'the appropriate' approach. The MCT was assumed to perform a reactive role in this respect. However, the officers considered the commissioning stage as the only phase in the ongoing management of local health services. This was seen as requiring the extensive involvement of the users, i.e. the health and unit administrators, because in this way the continuity in the provision of health care services could be ensured.

The MCT, just like any other team in the health service, were required to work on a 'consensus' basis. It was a mode described by DHSS circulars in terms of developing some 'common understanding' of the health service issues. An effective working relationship had thus to be established in order to facilitate the achievement of the targets and deadlines which were set in the management control plan. In most of their meetings the MCT for Newtown DGH reached agreement on various issues within the time-frame of the meeting. They argued strongly on certain issues and their impact upon the progress of the hospital project. Yet, they 'agreed to differ' and avoided any disagreement which could hinder the commence-ment of the construction activities and might be interpreted as disunity in the MCT. The minutes of the meetings, as the secretary of the meetings put it, were treated as 'action sheets'. They determined the activities of the members of the sub-groups. The minutes were the MCT's tribune and were used in their interactions with the members of the PT and the Newtown Development Corporation. They put the activities of the MCT members into acceptable and legitimate perspectives and sustained the momentum of the process of commissioning. The minutes reflected an adequate distribution of time to all items on the agenda. However, in the meetings, such issues as recruitment and training and revenue-cost consequences overshadowed health education, technology and public relations items. In setting these priorities the MCT could be seen as fol-lowing the 'Capricode' planning system, manpower planning followed the physical design of the hospital.

The agendas for the MCT meetings were prepared by the chairman. They followed a standard format and included a set of items regarding the tasks of the sub-groups and hence structured the discussions. The agenda was used by the chairman to sustain the momentum of the meetings, flow and continuity of the discussions. He controlled the amount of time which was spent on each item by interrupting or leading the discussions to the next item on the agenda. The participation of the members of the team in the meetings was fluid and varied with reference to the items on the agenda and different stages of the project development. For instance, at a time of financial crisis, the presence of the treasurers was more noticeable. Studies of such commissioning processes have often related the frequency of attendance to the motivation of the members of the commissioning team. They have described motivation in terms of intrinsic or extrinsic rewards which members seek individually to obtain. Thus the purpose of the process, i.e. the building of a new hospital, would be rewarding only if it fulfilled the actors' instrumental 'in-order-to' motives (as Schutz, 1967, described them). However, it is argued here that variations in attendance reduced the significance of the concept of 'team', i.e. a set of actors who worked together towards maintaining the continuity of health care provision, which was emphasized by the DHSS guidelines.

'Green field' sites and organization pre-histories

In the following section, the activities of the members of the MCT will be examined with reference to Miller and Rice's (1967) systemic model of organizational design. The model is chosen because it attempts to classify the staged process by which the design of both building and organizational structure take place on a green field site. It considers the extent of involvement of the actors and the way the task of design is interpreted and fulfilled by the actors within the context of established practices. It attempts to show that in the case of Newtown DGH the process of designing was heavily shaped by the 'Nucleus' assumptions set and popularized by the DHSS. Thus, the officers' claim that the green field site enhanced their choice options can be seen to be inadequately substantiated.

On the basis of Miller and Rice's model, the MCT for Newtown DGH could be described in terms of a 'temporary activity system'. A group of managers in the health service had been brought together to accomplish the task of building and commissioning a new DGH. The team would be dissolved when the task was completed since there would be no further *raison d'être* for the team. The MCT could be seen as an 'open system' responding to a set of environmental stimuli. The structure and functions of the team were formally devised on the basis of the task it was set up to accomplish. In accepting these delimitations, the actors identified boundaries which appropriated their approach to the commissioning of the DGH. Some of the actors had already commissioned previous large hospital buildings. They attributed significance to the particular characteristics of the planning and commissioning of Newtown DGH because it was being designed for and built on a 'green field' site. Accordingly, they emphasized the potential opportunities for establishing an innovative organizational culture within the well-established and traditional system of the NHS. However, their frame of reference contained the cultural and structural characteristics of various professions which operated within the old-established limitations of the NHS.

During the 1970s, as the ideology of managerialism grew in the NHS, the language of health care administration in the UK had developed an industrial vocabulary. Changes in the economic situation necessitated economies of scale in the NHS just like the mergers which took place in industry. The introduction of the 'Nucleus' hospital design indicated a movement towards efficiency cuts and savings, rationalization of resources and the use of cost-benefit analysis in the hospital projects. As a consequence, the frames and vocabularies of the team members and the type of building and organization design which the actors associated with the 'green field' site was profiled and adjudged with reference to this emergent set of new values. In particular the 'Nucleus' design 'Green Pack' was translated into drawings and parameters by the RHA designers and architects who were not the ultimate users nor were they involved in decisions about the allocation of resources. The 'Nucleus' planning/

building system more than ever determined the shape and use of space and resources in the minds of the RHA planners and designers.

The decision to build the hospital was initiated by Newtown Development Corporation and the senior officers of the DHA. Any further action would be outside the boundaries of their discretion because of its wide financial and organizational implications. Its location and timing were of political, economic and social concern and were thus dealt with by the officers at higher levels at the RHA and DHSS. This generated totally unpredictable time lags between various stages of the hospital project. In the case of Newtown DGH there was a 17-year period between the initial submission of the functional requirements of the new hospital, the preparation of design drawings and the actual construction of the building. Early in the process the MCT thought of leaving enough slack to adjust the operating systems during the construction process. However, the retiring District Nursing Officer perceived the process to be less smooth because he believed that

> the concept of [future] functional requirements would be out of date by the time it was constructed. [Moreover,] 'because people [could not] visualize changes . . . [the architects would] ask you what do you want? So you [would] describe the functional requirements . . . . Then later on you [would] play about with relationships, space in various departments. They [would] produce the first draft . . . . The users or planners [would] comment on it . . . etc.

Another of the planners reckoned that the actual physical design had only marginal effect on the staffing and the type of staff required. The main determinant would be patient workload.

The stages in project design suggested by Miller and Rice (1967) are as follows:

1 The design of the structure of the building: determining *what* physical resources and technology.
2 The design of the organization: determining *who* within human resources, what training for occupying the designed roles could be carried out in a parallel fashion.

In the case of DGH, planning followed this sequence. The design blueprint was there, so were the various groups of staff categories. The actors constructed and matched the organization and building structures of the DGH on the basis of anticipated future events. In principle the process should have ensured the integration of the activities of the staff and the resources. Yet, the workability of the designed operating system was as yet unknown.

In a situation of uncertainty the principal actors in the MCT shared the view of the nurse planner that 'Nucleus' standard design had provided them with 'pre-constructed operational objectives and policies' which in effect would determine the 'behaviour of the people'. The physical design was thus considered as the behaviour design and not just 'static drawings'. It was the means, for instance, for visualizing 'the movements of people' and examining the scope for alterations of dimensions. The commissioning experience of a previous DGH, its people and its problems constituted the 'quick reference', for those officers who had been working with the DHA and in the area for some years. Furthermore, the newcomers in the DHA had their own 'district specific' references about the relation between the hospital building and organization design. These references frequently altered their definitions and interpretations of their task boundaries. This cognitive process underlies Miller and Rice's more prescriptive model.

According to Miller and Rice's model, the design process is controlled through the defined physical and human requirements of the system which in essence reduces the need for any alterations in the later stages. The design of Newtown DGH on the basis of functional requirements was not a straightforward operation. Miller and Rice's model disregards the time lag that existed between the stages of (i) determining the functional requirements, (ii) translating these to the design of the building, (iii) interpreting these in its construction and (iv) commissioning the building and bringing into operational status. The complex composition of the MCT was however similar to that described by Miller and Rice as a 'management committee'. Thus it was made up of 'advisory groups', or subgroups which included membership of 'practitioners', some of whom were co-opted as convenors for the groups.

However, the authority relationships of members of the MCT followed the NHS hierarchy. Their membership of a temporary management organization did not extend their discretion or reduce their accountability. The involvement of the planners in the DHA in the design process was confined to their membership of the PT through whose machinery they introduced a number of modifications in the standard design package. They considered the design of the DGH as a technical matter which required their expert technical knowledge. The nurse planner was the only person who interpreted the design parameters, dimensions and conveyed the image of an operational reference for understanding the 'Nucleus' operating systems. Officers' visits to some completed 'Nucleus' projects also initiated reconsideration of some physical characteristics of the DGH. But the actors claimed that their manpower plan, i.e. organization design in Miller and Rice's terms, enhanced the chances of a successful commissioning and reduced the number of constraints which could not be anticipated. The 'Nucleus' standards had facilitated the integration of building and organizational design activities.

Stock of knowledge

Throughout the commissioning process, the MCT members worked on the design and planning issues whilst continually referring to:

- their own stock of knowledge as regards planning for a hospital
- the NHS-established patterns of thought and approaches
- 'Nucleus' standard design package
- various consultative and advisory documents provided by the DHSS and other research bodies which described the 'terms of reference' for the members of the MCT

All the members of the MCT and its sub-groups potentially had access to this stock of knowledge and knew their tasks and spans of discretion in the planning process. Their involvement in the process evolved within the boundaries of these guidelines. The terms of reference for the MCT included:

- 'network building' (Kotter, 1982), i.e. establishment of formal links with other teams and groups
- 'disseminating information', i.e. keeping the DMT informed about the difficulties and progress of the project
- 'coordinating' the interdependent activities and estimating the expenditure regarding different schemes
- 'selecting' an approach for handling any arising issue, thus
- 'seeking' to establish a united front

However, there were individual and local variations in the actors' earlier planning experiences within the NHS. Some actors played a supporting role in the process because they had had few planning experiences, or their previous experiences were in planning at the regional level which offered only a more distant overview with little contact with the individual hospital. All the principal actors claimed that their past experiences of commissioning hospitals justified their membership of the MCT and their role in the planning process. They suggested that their 'fairly wide knowledge of many elements that [went] into planning' had been developed over the years when there was no 'official reference'. They claimed that within the context of their experiences they were able to read architectural and engineering drawings and thus make contacts with the architects and works engineers to discuss the possible modifications in the standard design details.

It was a 'normal' situation for everyone who had worked for several years in the health services as a planner to become involved in the building of more than one hospital. Planning such services was seen as an inseparable element of the job. The knowledge that each had developed was the 'only salvation' that an officer had whilst climbing up the hierarchy. Without such experiences, the officers' 'comprehension of the health situation' would be limited. If they 'had the experience, their judgements could be of better quality'. It was like being in the army as the nurse planner put it,

> ... if you [had] an officer who'd come through and had some dirt under his finger-nails, at the end of the day he probably [would] be

able to make better value judgements than an officer who [had] been
to a military training school ... it [would be] the parcel of experience which [would] be beneficial to them.

Each officer's experience of commissioning of another district hospital was
soon to have a great impact upon their understanding of type and nature
of services which were considered for Newtown DGH and the problems
which they might face. Members remembered disastrous events from
previous commissionings. For example, it was discovered on one opening
day that the Audiology Department did not fit into the originally specified
requirements. Such re-adjustments were considered as typical and to a
certain extent predictable. These problems were also attributed to 'changes
in needs' that often the 'administrators and planners failed to compensate
for'. Staff characteristics and their performance in the existing hospitals
provided amendments to the 'Nucleus' 'formula' in Newtown DGH manpower plan.

These actors' familiarity with a range of NHS recipes for activities such
as capital planning turned the planning process into a morass of routine and mechanical considerations. DHSS guiding documents such as
'Preparing Manpower Plan' which explained the 'how' and 'what' of
approved human resource planning was such a constraint. There were no
documented or publicly announced sanctions for non-compliance of authorities to such set standards but approval of funds for different proposals
was linked to the extent that the formal norms had been incorporated.
The MCT developed an action plan in order to cope with the need for
tightness in the coordination of logistical administration and improve the
'quality of management decisions'. According to the nurse planner, this
approach worked because

in hard times people responded to it and there was security in it,
because they [were] told what to do. The instructions [were] clear,
measures and parameters [were] given ... just like the army. In the
army every day, every individual [would] read a piece of paper, i.e.
the agenda for the day.

The 'Nucleus' standard design pack provided the ultimate basis for this
agenda and thus the 'security' for the officers. Indeed the 'Nucleus' template contained the basic assumptions about what a hospital looked like
and what functional contents it should contain. In itself this basic template
mould reflected much of the NHS culture. But the team also developed
a set of shared mental constructs (Kelly, 1955). For example, a series
of phrases were repeated to describe the labour market, i.e. 'know your
people' meaning the identification of future staff and their interest groups.
Constructs also contained allusions to the risk of future disjunctures or
reconstruction of past events, i.e. for smoothing and extrapolation of
events. Other constructs had to do with setting 'action programmes and
timetables', etc. Thus, the critical path of events maintained a continuity

of action through their linguistic blending rather than a series of mechanistically discrete actions.

Intended discontinuity

Since the 'Nucleus' was a flexible planning and building system, the structuring and design of the organization of the DGH provided the officers with the desired leverage for 'breaking the mould' in the NHS. The actors often considered the *status quo* or 'continuity' in the context (i.e. political context) of their activities as a constraining element in the process of commissioning. They argued that 'the power [rested] with those who had the power for some while', i.e. 'the medics'. The MCT members searched for the ways in which they could 'change the existing power structure' in order to achieve their goals and beyond. As second-in-line officers they could not influence the selection of the medical staff, in particular consultants, for the hospital. They were not on the interview panel, because they had 'no power'.

> [The] Authority [had] no control over the consultants and the extent that they [were] using the resources (said the Administrators). Every consultant generated expenditure of £*x* million individually and yet they [were] not managed. Just like any other profession the Consultants' aim [was] to ensure they [were] paid by the state .... .

The MCT members thought of introducing certain sanctions into the DHA's staff rule-book for the new hospital which could be authorized by the DMT and would control the 'unacceptable' behaviour of medics to an extent. They argued that because Newtown DGH had got 'no hang-ups, no tradition, nothing, no culture' (i.e. a 'green field' site), they could create a novel situation where there were no 'lines of demarcation based on professionalism'. The personnel department thought that they could influence the process of recruitment by emphasizing the expenditure generated by the consultants' uncontrolled practices and their disagreeable professionalism. However, the popular belief among the officers was that 'you could not get anywhere if you tried simply to influence people by preaching that ... it is all for the efficiency of a hospital' or arguing that 'it is for saving the Authority's money'. That argument would fail. As the personnel manager put it, 'if you did go into the [negotiation] with just Taylor [i.e. Scientific Management] you'd get nowhere'. The alternative thus was 'to go in with some sort of human relations approach'.

The MCT agreed upon a gentle approach to the question of power because they believed that 'part of the resistance ... the initial armour was already broken' and 'once [they] created change in the culture' argued the nurse planner 'it did not matter what [target they] wanted to achieve'. Thus, as managers they were prepared to use themselves as 'change agents'. However, the question was to what extent their theorizing about domains of action and responsibilities within the future hospital organization and their speculations about the reactions of the professional groups to their plans created any more room for the achievement of their political goals? Their preferred situation, their ideal power structure, could only become a reality if their proposed staffing structure had been approved. Ultimately they had no authority to implement their proposed structures.

Conclusion

Membership of the MCT was like a 'power game' in which players attempted to change each other's positions, where and when they collectively perceived as appropriate. They held regular meetings to disseminate information about their perceived status in this game. When they assumed that they had gained the backing of the interest groups or their proposals were approved they announced that 'the ball [was] in [our] court' and that they were going to play it right. The common purpose attached to the MCT's actions was to ensure that the DGH was commissioned on time. Their publicly known reason for existence of the MCT enhanced the cooperation among its diverse membership. This was also necessary in order to fulfil their personal formal objectives, i.e. channelling the power relationships in their preferred direction. Thus, for the planners, the MCT meetings provided a continuing forum for airing their philosophies. Equally, it put pressure on them not to act outside this arena without the team's consensus. Their strategic activities evolved around the known rules in the commissioning process. It was understood that conforming to the group norms ensured the progress of the DGH and as the nurse planner put it 'there would be no frustration if one adjusted one's ideas' to such norms.

The explicit rules were dictated in the management control plan. Consequently, tasks were allocated to each member of the MCT and time deadlines were set for various schemes and planning activities. The actors' roles and responsibilities were clearly defined in the context of an hierarchy with varying degrees of discretion. In addition, there were some tacit rules in dealing with the environment of the group. For example, they were expected 'to accept the power of the medics' in the end. Actually, their repertoire of effective responses did not include any recipes with respect to reducing the power of the medics. They had developed a less aggressive approach to this group: their internal negotiations took place on a different note to that of other groups. Their main concern was to strengthen their network building activities and search to influence those groups who supported the DGH project in 'Newtown'. When their strategy was adversely affected by the delays in the construction activities their next move was to 'explain the facts' to the people and avoid 'spreading disappointment' among them. Their aim was to enhance the demand for a new DGH in the area by 'keeping everybody at it', as the general administrator described. The strategies which the MCT members adopted in the commissioning process served their collective and individual interests. If the hospital was built and commissioned according to their proposed plan the 'prestige' of Bordershire DHA would increase. All the officers in the DHA shared this belief. Equally, they assumed that their proposed modifications of the parameters in the hospital design package, their proposed training schemes and staffing structures (hence the hospital project as a whole) provided each of them with the 'vehicle for promotion': at the time of study some of the actors were indeed promoted to higher managerial levels.

Our observations illustrated the following characteristics of group activities in the commissioning process:

1 The recurrent nature of the work of a set of planners and administrators. Planning and design activities of the officers in the DHA were organized around a set of assumptions which the actors had developed within the 'cultural' values of the NHS and the context of administration and planning activities initiated and sustained by the DHSS, its design blueprint and manuals. The design blueprint had a structuring influence upon the activities of these actors. Therefore despite selection of a 'green field' site and the actors' perception of the novelty of the decisions the organizational characteristics of the DGH possessed pre-histories.

2 The planning activities included frequent 'mutual intellectual loading' by the actors and their role-set. The application of their 'interpretative schemes', which had developed accordingly, to their practices were considered as a routinized activity and sedimented in time. It is illustrated that these schemes simultaneously contributed to the very understanding and representation of their roles in the process of planning and design of a DGH.

3 The actors challenged established planning practices (the routinized side of their tasks) and proposed modifications of the details of hospital design, hence, attempted to reconstruct the power structure in relation to their role-set. They developed 'strategies' and 'rules' (within the same context) which provided them with some room for manoeuvre and thus the opportunity to transform and break the mould of the 'designed' approaches to planning for a DGH. Their transformational approach implied re-moulding of the context of their activities. The activities of these actors within their role-sets (i.e. medics, district officers) thus included their interventions into the 'present' in order to reconstruct the future. Faced with the ambiguity of decision making by the central resource allocators (DHSS and RHA) and lack of operational control over medical staff, the resultant outcomes seemed only to reproduce an existing equilibrium in the political system.

References

Kelly, J. (1955) *The Psychology of Personal Constructs*, Vol. I. New York: W.W. Norton.

Kotter, J.P. (1982) *The General Manager*. New York: Free Press.

Miller, E.J. and Rice, A.K. (1967) *Systems of Organisation*. London: Tavistock.

Schutz, A. (1967) *The Problem of Social Reality. Collected Papers. I.* The Hague: Martinus Nijhoff.

14 | Central Treatment: A Case of Smuggled Innovation

Margaret Grieco

Introduction

The preliminary concern of the research from which this chapter is drawn was with the possibility of the central direction of work organization and practice through the adoption of centralized and standardized hospital design.[1] In researching the relationship of workplace design to health work organization and work practice, two issues emerged as being of particular importance. Firstly, the relationship of workplace design to workplace organization and practice appears to be greatly affected or mediated by organizational culture. Secondly, the informal or interstitial power of nursing staff has been greatly underestimated in the conventional accounts of work organization and practice in the hospital setting.

In the course of the research reported upon here, the focus shifted away from a concern with the relationship between the physical and architectural aspects of workplace design and the centralized control of workplace organization towards an investigation of the micro-politics of the hospital context. The remainder of this chapter reflects this shift of interest. Before proceeding to a detailed discussion of this issue, it makes sense to indicate that our conclusion on the possibility of centralized or standardized hospital design as a mechanism for standardizing workplace practice is that such a tool is insufficient of itself to this purpose.

The nature of our preliminary research question led us to the selection of two identical hospitals as appropriate research sites. It is the selection and comparison of two identical hospitals which enables and permits the analysis of differences in organizational culture which follows the introduction. One of these hospitals is located in an East Anglian market town

– we refer to this as 'Market Town'. The other is located in London's green belt – we refer to this as 'Green Belt'. Within these hospitals, we focussed down upon the operation of one particular innovative design feature, the central treatment suite. The two cases examined here are both examples of the first UK standardized hospital design, termed 'Best Buy', and the introduction of the central treatment suite to UK hospitals first occurred as part of this design package.

The choice of the central treatment suite as the particular arena for investigation was informed by our prior research into health work organization and practice in a third area, a proposed standardized design hospital in a West Midlands New Town. In the course of investigating the politics of design of this West Midlands hospital our attention was drawn to an unheralded innovation in health practice, an innovation fostered by hospital designers attached to the central state agency and resisted and contested by the local agency responsible for health provision. This unheralded innovation was the adoption of central treatment rooms or suites as a routine feature of hospital design.

By unheralded innovation we mean to convey the extent to which the development and establishment of this practice has gone largely unannounced in the literature. The DHSS library has no document which details the development of this feature nor any document which explains its operation. The General Nursing Council neither announced its existence nor analysed its operation. Had our attention not been drawn to the existence of the central treatment innovation by this central–local dispute, it is unlikely that we would have been able to identify it by means of our literature review. Yet, we would argue, it is a key innovation in terms of hospital design.

Subsequent to our investigation of the design history of the West Midlands hospital, our researches focussed specifically upon the central treatment innovation. This interest has led us into an investigation of the source of the innovation, the sources of resistance to the innovation and the use or practice of central treatment in functioning hospitals.

Central treatment: policy contestation and smuggled innovation

Central treatment is a product of the attempted standardization and centralization of hospital design. Hospital construction pre-1950 was largely an *ad hoc* affair, though the Nightingale format provided the typical or standard template for ward design, much of the stock being a product of the Victorian sanitary boom. The 1950s, with the advent of the NHS, saw the standardization of technical detail with the introduction of hospital building notes and the regulation of hospital construction and design by central government. The late 1960s saw the expansion of activities on the part of the DHSS into the area of standardized hospital design. The DHSS to date has produced three standardized design packages: 'Best Buy', 'Harness' and 'Nucleus'.

The first of these, 'Best Buy', introduced the concept and practice of central treatment. The principle behind central treatment areas is that the dressing function, traditionally conducted on the ward, is now performed in a central location. The rationale provided for this change in the location of nursing tasks is twofold: firstly, central treatment, it is argued, reduces the risks of cross-infection, and secondly, the centralization of facilities reduces both capital and operational cost. The introduction of central treatment is also connected with the movement away from hostel provision for the sick towards short stay or early discharge treatment practices and the greater use of out-patient arrangements. Use of the central treatment area is controlled by an appointments system, the diminished flexibility on the timing of ward tasks being one important and obvious consequence of such a procedure. Armed with these preliminary and initial insights, we proceeded to investigate the practice of central treatment.

Our research on central treatment areas has taken two main directions. Firstly, we have documented the resistance to the principle in the West Midlands hospital – termed New Town – in some considerable detail elsewhere (Grieco, 1985a) and noted its apparent consequences in terms of developmental outcomes. To provide a brief summary, the evidence is that a complete rejection of the central treatment principle by the West Midlands planning team resulted in the considerable delay of the proposed hospital development. Resistance results, and is understood by those involved in the planning process to result, in delayed or aborted development. Secondly, we have, as already indicated, identified two identical hospitals – in different health regions – where the adoption of central treatment was not resisted at the level of physical planning, and have documented the nursing practices which have developed around the installation of this innovation in each hospital.

Senior staff in both these hospitals argued that in their opinion the uncontested acceptance of central treatment principles in the planning process was crucial to the rapid and positive outcome of the provision of the new hospital facility within both these locations. Within this chapter our concern is primarily with the second of these two lines of investigation, that is how the central treatment suite actually functions inside both hospitals. It should however be remembered throughout that resistance to the design feature of central treatment is not confined to the pre-provisionary planning period, as in New Town, but can occur in a variety of forms even where the facility has been installed without apparent resistance. The general point to be borne in mind is that there exists a widespread understanding that resistance to central design initiatives will result in delays in hospital provision and even threaten the prospect of any hospital development at all. The acceptance of whole hospital packages by medical and nursing staff takes place within a political and institutional environment where control rests primarily with the central government agency. In such a context, we can reasonably expect local adjustments to design intentions to occur.

Freedom of choice: a conceptual problem

Within this chapter, we argue that acceptance of the whole design package, and thus of central treatment, was in the case of Market Town and Green Belt a condition for the provision of the funds necessary for hospital construction. Unless central treatment was accepted, there would be no new hospital. The package was to be accepted completely: this was the only offer. In the case of the West Midlands hospital – hereafter called New Town – there was apparent freedom of choice. Rejection of the central treatment concept was an option and this option was exercised. The development which came into full use in February 1989, after a decade and a half of planning negotiations and activity, does not have central treatment rooms but does in fact have ward treatment rooms. The standardized design package, 'Nucleus', has been modified to meet the local requirements. However, given the extent of the delay to this to claim that there was simple freedom of choice is problematic, especially as hospitals which began their planning processes at the same time but followed the standard package template have enjoyed a substantially more rapid material translation from design to bricks and mortar.

Standardized design and differentiated practice: the role of organizational culture

Although the physical terrain of the two 'Best Buy' hospitals is identical there are considerable differences in the layout of the organizational terrain, so much so that the practices surrounding the use of the central treatment areas in one hospital are radically different from those adopted in the other. The evidence from this research is that even where green field organizational developments take place, and where the official stress is aggressively innovative, 'organizational cultures' frequently possess prehistories which are all too frequently left out of account in the literature (Grieco, 1988). The two hospital developments discussed in this chapter, although they were constructed simultaneously, emerged out of the rationalization of two entirely different health provision patternings.

The first hospital investigated – Market Town – represented a replacement for an old Victorian District General Hospital. Staff were merely transferred wholesale from one hospital to another. The second hospital investigated – Green Belt – contained centralized medical services which had previously been provided through ten separate cottage hospitals. These two hospitals diverged in their practices concerning the use of central treatment along a number of dimensions which reflect their previous organizational arrangements. For our purpose here, it serves to consider just two of these. In Market Town, where the founding staff was primarily drawn from the old District General Hospital, local general practitioners had no entitlement to the use of the central treatment suite for the performance of minor operations. In Green Belt, where the founding staff was primarily from the previous cottage hospital structure, general practitioners both had an entitlement and made substantial use of the central treatment suite for the conducting of minor operations. This practice represents a continuation of the previous and conventional cottage hospital practice where there were no resident medical staff. The absence of such a practice in Market Town is itself consistent with District General Hospital practice where resident medical staff compete for the control of hospital space. Under such circumstances, the provision of clinical space inside the hospital for general practitioners would be highly unusual. It should be noted that ironically the practice of providing general practitioners with access to the central treatment facility is highly consistent with present health policies of de-hostelizing health care but in fact emerges out of the more traditional of these two sets of health arrangements.

A similar divergence in practice between the two hospitals is to be found in portering arrangements. Because dressing and traumatic procedures are centralized within the 'Best Buy' design, patients have to be transported from the ward to the central treatment area for the conducting of procedures. This involves the substantial use of portering labour. Market Town, with its District General Hospital history, has a superior set of portering arrangements in terms of the availability of portering staff to the central treatment suite's nursing staff. The central treatment suite has its own porters at Market Town whereas at Green Belt the porters are allocated to the different sections of the hospital by the day. The central treatment unit at Market Town has an entitlement to two porters at any one point in time, whereas in Green Belt only one porter is allocated to the unit. At Green Belt porters are responsible for a number of clerical tasks in addition to the transporting of the patients between the central treatment suite and the ward, in Market Town the porters have upheld a strict and conventional definition of their task. In Market Town, the porters have established and maintained high manning levels in relation to the tasks performed. Two porters are required for the transportation of any one patient whereas in Green Belt the same task plus an additional set of tasks are performed by one man. Nursing staff in Market Town can request these portering teams to split in order to bring a greater number of patients into the central treatment area in particularly busy periods, but they can not insist upon it. The demarcation of tasks found in Market Town reflects the scale and the corresponding organizational and negotiating arrangements of such scale of the prior district General Hospital, the greater flexibility found in Green Belt reflects the more informal processes of work organization found in the Cottage Hospital structure.

The divergence of practice in two identical sites, subject to the same central policy direction, is, we argue, largely attributable to the carry over of practices from the old organizational structures into the new. This should not be taken to imply that the new sites and new designs have not resulted in any modifications to past practice, for indeed they have. We are merely attempting to establish the position that more care should be taken in the identifying of organizational pre-history and culture than is currently the vogue.

The relationship of the differences in practices between the two identical hospitals to the historical differences in the pattern of health provision between the two areas has been discussed more fully elsewhere (Grieco, 1985b). Our concern here is to introduce the notion that identical physical facilities do not of themselves determine the emergence of identical practices. Envelope does not determine practice, although it may indeed set certain of the limits.

At this point, we also wish to introduce the concept of resistance to a design innovation as being a dynamic which continues beyond the point of physical installation of a facility. In both the hospitals studied, resistance to central treatment innovation on the part of certain senior nursing personnel had persisted for over nine years. Installation did not ensure acceptance or comprehensive usage. Interestingly enough, precisely the nursing specialisms which were non-users in one hospital were the most allegiant users in the other, and vice versa. The persistence can largely be attributed to the territorial authority traditionally accorded the ward sister, which is to a large degree still retained in the present – although it has certainly been subject to encroachment at the margins.

In both hospitals, certain of the ward sisters categorically refused to countenance the use of the central treatment facility and indeed imposed a similar discipline upon the nurses serving under them. Furthermore, resistance to the use of central treatment areas was not confined to the ward sisters alone, for yet another pillar of resistance to the use of such facilities was to be found amongst consultants. Once again, resistance to the development was not to be explained by specialism, for those specialisms most resistant in one context, were the heavy users in another.

Traditionally, consultants inspected wounds more or less at will on their ward rounds. Inspecting a wound requires the re-dressing of a wound, yet the need to inspect a wound is not necessarily connected to any need for re-dressing *per se*. Thus traditionally the consultant's round was a major generator of dressing tasks. A properly used central treatment facility limits the consultant's autonomy over wound inspection considerably, for the appointment system operated in central treatment areas imposes a time-tabling discipline upon the consultant. Wound inspection becomes a highly programmed activity as compared with the traditional *ad hoc* or intuitive approach to the issue. Nursing sisters who favoured central treatment – in both hospitals – argued that the imposition of such a time-tabling discipline on consultants greatly reduced the volume of dressing traffic. Previously, they argued, wound inspection had been of little cost to the consultant but very expensive to the nursing staff in terms of the amount of additional work engendered. Central treatment was credited with generating a more responsible approach to wound inspection by consultants.

Yet, on other wards and in other specialisms in the same hospital, consultants and ward sisters formed alliances against the use of central treatment areas, precisely because they reduced the capability of both sister and consultant to inspect a wound at will. The installation of central treatment was perceived by some sisters as an instrument for extending autonomy *vis-à-vis* the medical profession whilst the very same facility was perceived by others as absolutely reducing the autonomy of the ward sister.

We have discussed, albeit briefly, complete resistance to an innovation at the level of physical planning in New Town: we have also discussed the continuing nature of resistance to a particular innovation and the organizational basis upon which such continuing resistance is viable. There is, however, an additional category to be placed on the continuum between complete resistance and complete acceptance of design innovations, and that is the category of local design modification.

In both of the cases we have examined, acceptance of the standard design with its incorporated central treatment facility was a pre-condition of hospital provision. In both areas, the new hospital was urgently required. Thus outright organizational resistance to the facility was not a viable option. The space for negotiation at this point in the design history of both developments was highly restricted, with real sanctions lying in the balance. A subsequent and continuous pressure for modification is, however another matter, the threat of no development having already been neutralized. Neither hospital has had any opportunity to feed these complaints and recommendations into the on-going DHSS design programme on standardized hospital construction. There have been no formal linkages between the users and the designers beyond the commissioning period. Nor have any other relevant agencies contacted these pioneers in order to investigate emerging design and usage problems.

Nevertheless, modification of the facilities by the users is indeed taking place in both locations. Indeed, some of the same modifications have been made on both sites without any coordinating agency being involved and in the absence of contact between the two sets of personnel. For instance, alarm bells have been installed inside the treatment rooms in both sites as the consequence of similar crises in patient care. Because of the desire to provide privacy in the treatment rooms, events within these rooms are not visible from outside. Without an alarm bell, and where a solitary nurse is present, where a patient is in crisis, i.e. a heart attack, the nurse is unable to summon help without endangering the patient. The occurrence of the same type of event in both locations led to the same resolution, the failure to provide this facility in the first instance can be regarded as a major design failure. In both sites, the bulk of modifications appears to be accomplished through in-house bargaining between departments rather than through any external bargaining with the central authorities responsible for design. This, of course, has the consequence that bad design is not receiving the necessary feed back to correct its inadequacies, and indeed we pick this point up elsewhere (Grieco, 1985c) in the discussion on technical versus democratic rationales for participation in the design process.

To summarize, within this section, we indicated that the two hospitals which pioneered the central treatment concept in a UK context were poorly placed to resist the innovation. In both cases, the health authorities concerned were offered a package which they had either to accept or to reject wholesale. Refusal would have resulted in the failure to provide any new facility whatsoever. It is in this sense that we term central treatment a smuggled innovation, for there was no space for discussion on the acceptability of its arrival. It was imposed from above without consultation with the relevant users. Furthermore, the innovation remains largely undiscussed, as do its implications for nursing practice and work organization.

Resistance to the innovation has taken a number of forms, the most relevant of which to our present discussions is that of discretionary non-use in the context of organizational use – that is to say, hospital policy and ward sister policy are at odds – and in-house design modifications. We noted that the central treatment facility may be used by nursing staff as an instrument for extending their autonomy over medical staff, but that it may also be resisted as an encroachment upon the territorial authority of the ward sister, and that alliances may form between consultants and ward sisters in order to preserve the traditional territorial boundaries which threaten to be disrupted by the central treatment innovation.

This alliance concerned with the preservation or re-establishment of the old *status quo* is not the only alliance formed between senior nursing staff and senior medical staff around the provision of central treatment facilities. Indeed, in both hospitals a competitive treatment policy existed between consultants around the annexing of central treatment facilities for specialist clinics. Furthermore, nursing staff possessed discretionary authority around the time-tabling of central treatment use in both locations. Alliances between the central treatment staff and particular specialists were crucial in determining the functioning of the units. Elsewhere (Grieco, 1985d) we compare the weekly timetable of the two units, paying attention both to the official statistics and to official nurse management policies, and to the unofficial dimension of activities as identified through participant observation. To provide a simple example, the nursing sister in Market Town frequently permitted the 'scopes' consultant use of the treatment facility beyond his official quota. In doing so she was operating against the express instructions of the nursing officer who was attempting to restrict the consultant's use of the facility in order to obtain the leverage necessary, by the creation of a usage crisis, to increase the financial resources available to the unit.

In the next section we confine ourselves in the main to the practices and characteristics of Market Town hospital. This was the first of two developments to be visited, and serves as a useful introduction to the whole case.

Market Town: demonstration centre and self-conscious pioneer

In examining the central treatment area at Market Town we are examining a pioneer development. But we are actually analysing much more than that, for the central treatment area here operates very much as a demonstration centre or show place. Potential users of the 'Best Buy' package or indeed of the other packages which host the central treatment area are directed to this site by the experts at the (former) DHSS in order to observe the concept at work. Visiting traffic to the development is heavy indeed – much of it British, but with a fairly generous sprinkling of visitors from overseas interested in purchasing design packages and construction expertise. The unit is, not surprisingly, practised at receiving visitors, though mainly these are of the 'day trip' rather than the extended stay variety.

Here there is a rather neat but discrete anthropological point to be made. The unit had a whole repertoire and coordinated account of itself with which it furnished the day visitor (Pettigrew, 1979). This account minimized the real problems and hiccups experienced in administering the unit to a considerable extent (Grieco, 1988). The account provided by the same actors during the period of participant observation was radically different. Problems are more disguisable in relation to the casual or passing visitor than they are in relation to the practitioner, be they transient or permanent.

Entering Market Town as a casual visitor in the first instance, and negotiating fuller access after this visit, permitted the collection of contradictory accounts from the same personnel in a manner that would not have been possible using any other approach. The same approach was used for Green Belt, it should be noted, although the different mode of organization in this location rendered it difficult to conceal administrative hiccups even from the most casual of visitors. For instance, because porters at Green Belt were despatched for patients before treatment rooms became free, any fall back in the treatment programme resulted in patients queueing, in their beds and wheelchairs in the reception area of the central treatment suite. Thus any fall back in the treatment programme became visible as corridor congestion. In Market Town, strict adherence to the central treatment principle of reducing the potential for cross-infection meant that porters were only despatched for patients when a treatment room became free. Thus whilst fall backs in treatment programme occurred as frequently in Market Town as they did in Green Belt, because of different patient transportation arrangements such disruptions in the schedule were not immediately visible.

However, the same general principle of best face forward to the casual visitor also held true at Green Belt. Visitors were not however the rule at Green Belt. Whereas Market Town has been fostered as a demonstration centre, Green Belt has not. What are the implications of labelling an organization or unit a show place? In Market Town the apparent consequence of such a status is the high levels of commitment of staff to the unit. The staff of this unit are particularly innovative and technology conscious, as compared with their counterparts at Green Belt. A consciousness of innovativeness permeates the 'organizational climate' of the unit, a consciousness which is consistent with unit policy of seconding nurses to external technical training schemes run by medical equipment suppliers. No such policy of secondment of nurses to external training schemes exists at Green Belt.

Our argument, put simply, is that show centre status feeds, reinforces and maintains the consciousness of innovation and is productive of other innovatory behaviours (Lilja, 1988; Rasanen and Kivisaari, 1988). This innovatory consciousness is, however, very much a one-sided phenomenon, for the nursing staff of the Market Town unit had never visited another functioning central treatment area. Furthermore, at the time of fieldwork they had never considered doing so. This, despite the fact that they knew of a number of hospitals presently operating a central treatment facility. Our point here is that the consciousness of innovation present in Market Town was not accompanied by any systematic search or process of comparison which would permit the determination of best practice.

We have stressed the extent to which the unit is innovation conscious on account of its show place status and its associated exposure to admirers, but there is yet another process which further fosters such a consciousness, that is the use of the central treatment area staff as an induction agency in hospitals which are about to commence on the central treatment format.

The team is used not only as a source of technical expertise but also as an agency of persuasion. The team visits hospitals where central treatment facilities are to be installed and fields a panel to discuss the system with the nursing establishment. The team, needless to say, is composed of the positively inclined with respect to central treatment concepts – and indeed it is to be noted that day visitors to Market Town itself are only put into contact with adherents to the system. Typically the team expects and receives a rough ride in such situations, the concept of central treatment being as it is at variance with the concept of total patient care introduced into health care by the General Medical Council in the 1960s. Central treatment fragments the nursing task, removing a major source of job satisfaction from the ward (Grieco, 1985e).

To place an innovation framework around this general set of points, pioneer status ensures the continuation of positive attitudes towards the innovation, the pioneer status of the establishment being the basis of intense and continuing attention. Here we are suggesting that there is a relationship between show place status and continued commitment to a particular form of organization. One interesting speculation arising out of this particular line of thought concerns the well-publicized socio-technical systems developed by Rice in Ahmedabad. The pioneer development retained a health not possessed by other such developments. It is pertinent to enquire whether pioneer status of itself invoked the necessary commitment for the continued functioning of such as an experiment.

Although we will not attempt to develop the argument on the re-lationship between show place status and expressions of satisfaction with technical and organizational innovation any further here, it does seem to us to be a point of some general importance or significance for any sociological account of the diffusion process.

In the case of Market Town, there is a special feature of commitment to the experiment of pioneer status which deserves our attention. Experi-mental status was imposed upon Market Town. As no discussion was permitted as to the form the development would take, no arguments had to be advanced. Design became reality without any associated articulation of principles. Adherence to central treatment in Market Town was therefore an adherence to practice, not an adherence to principle, in the first instance. Elsewhere (Grieco, 1985e), we have discussed, for example, the extent to which the training and recruitment procedure at Market Town generates commitment as a consequence of the failure to discuss alternatives.

Resistance and practice: the role of skirmishing

Resistance to the central treatment concept in the New Town case origin-ated with the nurse planning officer based at the Area Health Authority. He successfully advanced, researched and articulated the case against cen-tral treatment areas. Our research into the use of central treatment areas would have progressed significantly more slowly without the benefit of his clear and lucid argumentation as to the disadvantages of central treat-ment areas. His argumentation contained both technical and professional strands, the professional was however fairly heavily cloaked in a technical dressing throughout the debate.

The strength of feeling exhibited by this officer around the issue, we read to be most probably typical rather than unique, and indeed when presented initially with such a monolithic, pro-central treatment perspec-tive in Market Town, we decided to widen the basis of our sample.

The Market Town unit staff tried to a large extent to preclude contact with the dissenters, even once research had moved onto a participant observation basis. The chief nursing officer in particular spent some considerable time attempting to guide the direction of the interview schedule outside of the unit. There were, however, advantages to be had by the researcher from the central treatment appointments system and method of record keeping. Non-users of the facility were immediately identifiable from a quick scan of the data sheets; low use rates on the part of any particular ward signalled the location of pockets of resistance.

Central direction of design does not, it seems, within the current rules of the game, result in the central direction of practice. Non-use of the facility is not attributable to technical factors *per se*, for not only is it the case that the specialist pattern of usage in Market Town is the reverse image of the specialist pattern of usage in Green Belt, but it is also the case that within the Market Town site alone, a change of ward sister frequently signals a change in approach to the central treatment facility. Resistance to the facility, as we have already noted, remained past the period of installation. Indeed, such resistance remains even where majority nursing opinion within the hospital is pro-central treatment.

Interaction between the nursing managers in alliance with central treatment staff and dissenting sisters can be characterized as consisting principally of skirmishes around the extent of the sister's authority. Thus when a dissenting ward sister is off duty, central treatment staff host nurses and patients from the ward in the prohibited central space. Nurses experiencing an overload of dressing work will, in the absence of the dissenting sister, send their patients to central treatment.

Blow-ups over such subversion of ward practice and sister's authority appear to be quite common, though not normal events. Our evidence on such skirmishes is, however, reported rather than observed, although during the period of fieldwork the 'kidnapping' of patients from the ward to central treatment was witnessed, happening in the ward sister's absence.

The social segregation of dissenters appeared to be a powerful dynamic. Interestingly, dissenters were to be found in pairs, that is to say they were sisters on adjacent wards. Such adjacency provides for easier contact and presumably permits the value reinforcements necessary to resistance in this skirmishing environment.

One of the New Town rationales for the rejection of the central treatment area was that it precluded the sister's monitoring of patients' progress, and indeed of the nurses' progress as well. Central treatment reduces the importance of the sister, both in respect of her nursing, training and general supervisory functions. These technical objections can, as we have already indicated, be converted into terms of authority and territory; central treatment areas undermine the authority and power base of ward sisters.

The installation of central treatment facilities was accompanied by other design changes which can be viewed as altering the ward power base of sisters. The major alteration of importance from this perspective is that of ward form or layout. The old Nightingale wards – a design which was discussed with nostalgia and fondness by all – provided the sister with a windowed office which permitted a full view of the ward but which also offered a considerable degree of privacy in respect of sound.

The current design has moved the sister's office off the ward, thus rendering the simultaneous conduct of confidential conversations and ward supervision impossible. The current vogue for bays – separated by permanent screens – heightens the problems involved in sister's supervision of both patients and nurses. The Victorian 'pan-optic' template for ward design has been abandoned.

Furthermore, this design generates major problems with traffic flow, coupled as it is to the central treatment facility. For with central treatment, beds are routinely moved about the hospital from ward to central dressing area and back to ward. Central treatment means the circulation of a great number of beds down alleyways and corridors in spaces which are poorly designed to accommodate such traffic. These features of design would seem to indicate a lack of acquaintance with nursing tasks, and are clearly evidence of insufficient user feedback. Design issues apart, what is clear is that the combination produced within the standard hospital packages reduces the supervisory capability of the ward sister directly.

The central direction of practices: obstacles and diversions

Nursing practice and nursing standards were at the point of research governed by the General Nursing Council (GNC). The GNC routinely visited hospitals on an annual basis and checked that the standard of training and the standard of practice fell within its general guidelines. It had considerable power, for it was legally able to withdraw nurses from wards which it regards as inadequately staffed, and thus effectively has the power to close wards down completely.

As we indicated in the introduction, the GNC provided no particular or general guide to the operation of central treatment facilities. Their operation is initially authored by the individual hospitals involved – thus the practices pertaining in Market Town both with regard to normal use and training use are substantially different to those followed in Green Belt. The hospital did not, however, have complete control over its operational policy, for the GNC had a veto over any nursing practice which it regards as unsatisfactory. Within the Market Town hospital, the GNC found no fault with the present nursing practices surrounding central treatment. Indeed, the issue has never been discussed as such.

The situation in Green Belt is, however, radically different. Here the GNC expressed extreme displeasure with the existing arrangement. Indeed, there have been protracted negotiations throughout the life of the hospital between the GNC and the nursing managers of Green Belt. The hospital's initial policy on central treatment had been substantially modified by the GNC' explicit recommendations. The point to note here is that any change is accomplished on a hospital-by-hospital basis without any explicit theorizing or general codification. Each hospital operates in ignorance of the practices adopted in other hospitals. Information on the practices utilized in other hospitals is generated via the mobility of labour rather than by any other path; thus sisters arriving from other regions carry information on different practices with them. The GNC represents a rather limited agency of diffusion.

Sisters could, however, rely on a certain level of protection from the GNC in their adherence to traditional practices. Thus there exist two important sources of policy direction on nursing tasks: that is, hospital policy and ward policy. Hospital policy, we would argue, is more amenable to central direction, lying as it does largely in the hands of hospital administrators, than is ward policy, which lies largely within the control of the nursing sister. Ward policy can, at least on the evidence of Market Town, override hospital policy. The suspicion is that over time, however, such pockets of resistance will die out as sisters are appointed who have trained within a central treatment regime.

A further point to be noted at this stage is that the existence of central treatment areas does enhance the role of nursing officers as distinct from ward sisters – for nursing officers have more powers of direction over central treatment senior nursing staff, i.e. departments, than they do over ward staff. Ward sisters appear, at least on the evidence of Green Belt and Market Town, to have control over all that happens within their defined territory – patients belong to the ward and relationships are relatively fixed, whereas on departments, patients are essentially borrowed. The relationship of patient ownership to territory appears within both these hospitals to be a factor of some considerable importance. We have searched the literature for an analysis of this relationship, but to date it remains undiscussed. To put the point differently, departmentalizing nursing tasks reduces absolute nursing power. Central treatment, we are emphasizing, by its very nature owns no patients; furthermore, where its use is widespread, it has the direct consequence of limiting the ownership of patients by the ward.

Whereas within Green Belt, the presence of trained staff other than central treatment staff was itself rare, in Market Town the central treatment area experienced transient staff, i.e. staff from the wards, passing through its working space at a very high frequency. Where this is the case, the presence of outsiders over whom the sister has no control is large. This departmental situation represents a direct contrast with the situation on the wards. Some of the difference between Market Town and Green Belt on the prevalence of outsiders in the departments' working space is explained by different training systems, and some by different operational policies. Despite the attempt to introduce standardized structures, different policies, practices and patterns still prevail in structurally identical sites.

Within the hospital sector, then, we argue, policy is more important in determining practice than physical structure. Furthermore, local policy differences continue to be important within the same central policy framework. We note that hospital policy, during the period of the research, was formulated within the context of a powerful GNC, an institution which could considerably strengthen the power of senior nursing staff in their defence of traditional authority relations. The GNC did not always serve as a support to the nursing interest, it may indeed have been antagonistic towards any particular hospital nursing staff's preferred mode of procedure. It is precisely this situation which has occurred in Green Belt. Although it is dangerous to generalize on the basis of but two examples, it does seem to be the case from the evidence we have collected, that the GNC demonstrated more of a conservative than a progressive bent in terms of its orientation towards nursing practice. Market Town was not subject to the same exacting process of censure as was Green Belt, for Market Town was still operating within the general framework of total patient care, at least on paper, even within the limitations imposed by the presence of a central treatment area.

Innovation or anachronism?: changes in nursing practice and their consequences for the use of central treatment areas

The manner in which central treatment areas should be used is however an area of contestation for reasons other than those advanced in the previous section. For at more or less the same time that architects were designing facilities which would rationalize dressing tasks, nursing and medical practices were changing in a direction which substantially reduced the need for the facility.

At the point of commencement of design of central treatment areas, it was general medical practice to dress wounds daily and to follow such a regime for some considerable time after the operation had taken place. Furthermore, at this point in time the normal duration of stay in hospital was significantly longer than was later to become the case. The early records of central treatment area usage in Market Town evidence high initial rates of dressing traffic which declined quite rapidly in the late 1970s.

This appears to indicate that central treatment only served its intended function during the early stages of development, for past this point, although it continues to be used for dressing traffic, it begins to take on the character of host to special clinics. Although our resources did not stretch to coding the data held by Market Town on its past, it was made available to us and we were able to scan the information presented on the thousands of data sheets held, but never analysed. We were thus in a position to form a fairly accurate impression of the changes which had taken place, and this fitted with actors' accounts. In the case of Green Belt, such information had not been retained, although the nursing staff furnished much the same account.

Shortly after the introduction of central treatment areas, changes in practice associated with wound dressings occurred; wounds which were previously dressed are now left exposed, coupled with the advent of early discharge policies which significantly lessened the volume of custom for hospital dressing services, as patients were receiving an increased proportion of their treatment at home where nursing was provided by community nurses. Furthermore, early discharge reduced, it is argued, the incidence of cross-infections and this in its turn also reduced the demand for dressings. Thus it would seem that central treatment areas were introduced to rationalize a specific set of needs which have now apparently disappeared, or at least in their most acute form.

In both Market Town and Green Belt, a certain volume of dressing traffic continues, but these dressings are largely associated with traumatic procedures, e.g. colonoscopies, bed sores, catheterization, etc. rather than with routine dressing of surgical wounds. Central treatment continues, according to the nursing staff, to have a function in such circumstances as the following: it provides the patient with a privacy that is difficult to provide on the ward, and protects other patients from unnecessary anxieties. Elsewhere (Grieco, 1985f) we have discussed patients' perceptions and preferences around the use of central treatment areas; here we wish only to signal that whereas the central treatment area may have lost utility in terms of volume of dressings, it retains some specialist functions.

Within Market Town competition exists amongst senior medical staff for the use of and control over the central treatment facilities. The competition for control of these facilities is, however, subject to the rules imposed by senior nursing staff. Comment already abounds in the literature as to the virulence of competition amongst consultants for bed, and, consequently, ward space. The competition for central treatment facilities precisely parallels this process, for in the same fashion that the control over beds provides the consultant with control over his workload and workflow, control over central treatment facilities provides him with the same quality of discretion over day- and out-patients.

It should be noted at this point that both Market Town and Green Belt central treatment facilities are extensively used in the treatment of private patients. Private patients represented a greater proportion of the patient traffic in Green Belt as compared with private usage in Market Town during the respective periods of field study. Although private/NHS patient differences are not entered on the permanent record sheets, nursing staff in both locations said that the ratio observed during the fieldwork period was the normal one.

Central treatment facilities have, over time, become primarily used for minor operations rather than for dressing tasks, although this was not originally intended to be the case. Consultants have more ready access to the central treatment operating rooms than they have to the operating theatres.

The major medical contenders for central treatment time and space are the consultant surgeons, eye surgery, tube surgery (colonscopes, gastroscopes) and vasectomies being the predominant specialisms. There is a strong overlap between the specialist functions performed in Market Town central treatment area and Green Belt central treatment area, but it is not a complete replication of procedures. For instance, Green Belt central treatment area is the venue for electro-convulsive therapy, a somewhat controversial practice used in the treatment of long-term depression whereas Market Town is not. Some measure of the present extent and virulence of controversy around this issue is provided by the knowledge that this was the only procedure conducted in Green Belt central treatment area in which central treatment staff took no part.

Viewed slightly differently, the electro-convulsive therapy clinics were the only occasions on which the central treatment staff were required to relinquish their control over the use of facilities. This clinic had an entitlement to two sessions a week, and unless more time was required, the psychiatric staff had no need to negotiate their position with central treatment. Furthermore, it is in the nature of such treatment that its use is highly predictable in character – it is not an emergency procedure; rather its use is dictated by chronic conditions. Whereas those involved in conducting emergency procedures are highly dependent upon the aid of central treatment staff in time-tabling, scheduling and allocating space for these activities, planned and predictable use of the facility carries no such inherent dependence on the grace and favour of central treatment staff.

Scanning central treatment records for Market Town, we noted that during the late 1970s and at the very beginning of the 1980s, central treatment facilities had been used for conducting abortions. These abortions had involved the use of prostaglandin rather than surgical methods, with the use of prostaglandin being noted on the record sheets. Initially we thought that these central treatment area procedures might be part of a national experiment orchestrated by the John Radcliffe Hospital, Oxford, where major research on the use of prostaglandin as an abortion technique was being conducted in the same period.

In the context of interviewing nursing staff at Market Town as to the policy change in the venue of abortions, it emerged that prostaglandin abortions were perceived as primarily being given to teenage girls with the intention of providing a lesson to them. The consultant responsible fully realized the unpleasant character of prostaglandin as an abortion technique as compared with that conducted under general anaesthetic. However, in order to stop girls using abortion as a form of birth control, prostaglandin was deliberately used to render the experience unpleasant and thus reduce repeat demands for abortions.

Using the prostaglandin technique places a greater demand on nursing staff while simultaneously reducing the workload of consultants, for under this technique hormones are introduced intravenously to the body, encouraging induced labour. This process does not require a consultant's presence; it is however like labour, a process which can be of considerable duration and requires, as such, high levels of nursing attention.

Central treatment staff were, it should be noted, not obliged to participate in these procedures, but often did so. Those staff interviewed upon this topic registered a strong dislike of the practice as it had occurred, viewing the discomfort engendered in these teenage girls as unnecessary and pointless, although declaring themselves as having no moral objections to abortion *per se*. Abortions, like electro-convulsive therapy, are an area of medical practice subject to considerable controversy and the voluntary character of unit staff participation in this procedure reflected the more general state of play on the national scene.

Central treatment space afforded these two highly traumatic procedures a high level of screening from general observation in the hospital environment. In the case of electro-convulsive therapy, the treatment is short in duration and treatment rooms are freed from use within a relatively fixed interval. In the case of the prostaglandin abortions the duration of the treatment is lengthy and unpredictable, freezing rooms from other usage for some considerable time. The latter factor, taken in combination with competition for the use of the facilities for minor purposes, appears to provide the rationale for the decline in the number of abortions performed within the unit.

Central treatment, time-tabling and the enhancement of nursing power

As already implied by the various references to competition, not all consultants share the same access to the central treatment area; there are indeed differential qualities of access. Some consultants are able to schedule minor operations at will, whilst others attempting to secure the equivalent allocation of time and space may be effectively blocked by the central treatment staff, for the nursing staff have overall responsibility for the scheduling, time-tabling and general running of the central treatment area. Nurses are able to arrange timetables so as to thwart consultants' intentions.

It is not easy to assess how consistently such thwarting took place of the same consultants but the organizational myths were to the effect that this could and indeed did take place. We were however in a position to witness a number of obstructive events which supported this claimed competence. Our point here, then, is that the reduction of demand for dressing space resulted in spare capacity existing within the central treatment areas. This spare capacity induced competition amongst the various medical specialisms for control of the space. The nursing staff occupied a pivotal position in their responsibility for the timetable of the central treatment suite and this provided them with a form of informal or interstitial power (Grieco and Whipp, 1986; Rosser and Davies, 1986). Where a consultant or junior doctor required access to the facility on an unscheduled basis, this further enhanced the informal powers of the nursing staff. For whereas a doctor could with the benefit of a lengthy bargaining period obtain the necessary scheduling of central treatment space against a predictable set of demands, the need for immediate accommodation in unpredictable circumstances increases the dependency on the central treatment staff.

Thus whilst in general central treatment staff were subject to the power of the medical staff, there were particular moments in which this relationship was reversed, albeit informally and fragmentarily. It is as a consequence of the existence of such moments of power that coalitions are developed between particular consultants and the central staff, with such consultants playing a role in the recruitment of nursing staff sympathetic to their cause.

Conclusion

The object of this chapter has been to argue that the central design of workplace does not, of itself, result in the central control of work organization and practice. Even where organizations appear to be 'green field' in character, previous organizational histories and forces are in play which serve to produce differences in the practices and patterns between one location and another. The chapter has argued that nurses' powers of resistance and control to imposed developments frequently take an informal character and have gone largely unrecognized in the existing literature. It also argued that insufficient attention is paid to nursing knowledge in the hospital design process. New Town hospital's design history represents the exception.

The introduction of central treatment suites on the evidence available would seem to reduce the power and authority of one group or section of nurses, ward sisters, whilst increasing the power and authority of another, central treatment specialist staff. Whilst, in the present, resistance to central treatment practices remains a significant factor, with time and the turn over of older nursing labour, resistance is likely to weaken and central treatment practices will become increasingly accepted and go uncontested. Central treatment practices are, however, likely to vary between sites under the influence of the complex of organizational factors and practices within which they themselves are located.

Note

[1] The research on which this chapter is based was undertaken as part of the Work Organisation Research Centre Programme, University of Aston, 1982–7. This chapter was revised and completed as Visiting Scholar, Lucy Cavendish College, Cambridge.

References

Grieco, M.S. (1985a) *The Politics of Hospital Design: The Freedom to Modify, the Power to Veto* (mimeo). Work Organisation Research Centre, University of Aston.

Grieco, M.S. (1985b) *Organisational Culture and Green Field Sites: The Power of Past Patterns of Organisation and Association* (mimeo). Work Organisation Research Centre, University of Aston.

Grieco, M.S. (1985c) *Designing in Bad Practice: The Need for Greater Consultation in Hospital Design* (mimeo). Work Organisation Research Centre, University of Aston.

Grieco, M.S. (1985d) *Informal Power and the Construction of Crisis: The Development of Leverage in the Negotiating Process* (mimeo). Work Organisation Research Centre, University of Aston.

Grieco, M.S. (1985e) *Central Treatment and the De-skilling of Ward Nurses* (mimeo). Work Organisation Research Centre, University of Aston.

Grieco, M.S. (1985f) *Emotional Work, Technical Locale: The Role of the Nurse in Reducing Patient Anxiety* (mimeo). Work Organisation Research Centre, University of Aston.

Grieco, M.S. (1988) Birthmarked: A critical view on analysing organisational culture. *Human Organisation*, **47**(1), 84–7.

Grieco, M.S. and Whipp, R. (1986) Women and the workplace: Gender and control in the labour process. In: *Studies in Gender and Technology in the Labour Process*, Knights, D. and Wilmott, H. (eds). Gower: Aldershot.

Lilja, K. (1988) *Organisational Learning in the Contexts of Managerial Work: The Case of the Kaskinen Pulp Mill*. Working Paper 88–12. European Institute for Advanced Studies in Management.

Pettigrew, A. (1979) On studying organisational cultures. *Administrative Science Quarterly*, **24**, 570–81.

Rasanen, L. and Kivisaari, S. (1988) DAMATIC and its extending dimensions: a description of managerial work in a case of corporate innovation. In: *Workshop on the Study of Managerial Labour Processes, European Institute of Advanced Studies in Management, May, 1988*.

Rosser, J. and Davies, C. (1986) Gendered jobs. In: *Studies in Gender and Technology in the Labour Process*. Knights, D. and Wilmott, H. (eds). Gower: Aldershot.

15 | The Future of Health Care Delivery – Markets or Hierarchies?

Ray Loveridge

This volume began with a paradox. It posed the question of why, in one of the few areas of organized activity in which the UK service providers remain world class performers, the Thatcher Government felt impelled to introduce radical reform. The question was made more insistent by both the intention and mode of innovation adopted by that administration in the Health Service Act of June 1990 and in the series of reports through which reform has been initiated over the preceding decade. Taken together these amount to the creation of competition between different units of the NHS for the custom of the primary carers, and ultimately in some cases, that of the patient. The answer found by Cox in Chapter 2 was that of an ideological distaste for communal action of the kind incorporated in the original design of the NHS. Quite clearly the 1990 Act was an extension of the Thatcherite belief in the unregulated workings of the market as the most effective means to allocate resources efficiently. Within this logic the continuation of the NHS as a publicly financed and centrally administered service might seem unlikely to remain unchallenged. According to many observers we might therefore anticipate possible future steps on the road to the privatization of health care under possible Conservative administrations (Pollitt et al., 1988).

By way of contrast, on the day that the internal market was introduced into the UK NHS the French Government was agreeing a system of statutory health service subscriptions with the three national medical interest associations in that country not dissimilar to the original Beveridge proposals for the NHS. In the USA a wide range of leading employers including AT&T, Ford, Eastman Kodak, General Electric, Lockheed and Xerox began the new decade by creating a unique coalition behind a concerted campaign under the title of National Leadership Coalition for Health Care Reform. Medical costs were seen to be increasing at more than double the general inflation rate while private employers were shouldering approximately 28 per cent of direct health costs through employee contributions to private insurance schemes (Kuttner, 1991). What divided this influential coalition were issues such as how comprehensive any possible government mandated alternatives to a mixed economy in health care should be and what should be the extent of the tax-supported element. What united these corporate employers was an apparent belief that the care providers, including the pharmaceutical and equipment suppliers and the health insurance agencies, were united in an informal cartel to 'gold-plate' the treatment on offer and to complicate billing in order to disguise the true costs of care delivery.

Clearly it is no coincidence that the economics of health care should be the subject for national debates across most industrialized countries at this time. Over a prolonged period of economic crisis most industrial states have sought to rationalize and retrench their investment in social welfare. As Starkey has suggested in Chapter 4 economic contingencies have brought about increased attempts at greater administrative control over state employees throughout the preceding decade; most particularly this has been so in direct services such as education and health care in which considerable autonomy have hitherto been enjoyed in the task of service delivery. Nor should it necessarily be surprising that strategic responses should differ so drastically. Governments have adopted strategies deriving from the historically unique relationships existing within their countries between the professional institutions and the state. These have both acted on, and been shaped by, the broader ideological stance adopted by political administrations toward the provision of the core services of education and health care, within each nation over a long period (Child and Loveridge, 1990).

Dimensions of control and autonomy

As has been demonstrated throughout this volume, the influence exercised by health care professionals at the point of production is almost certainly greater than that available to service deliverers in any other sector of employment. Equally the effect of occupationally imposed hierarchy has been present even where, as in the process of commissioning of new hospital buildings described by Sharifi (Chapter 13), it has been felt in the physical absence of medical consultants. In this sense the unconscious framing of strategic agendas around professional templates provides an extension of their workplace authority into the formation of long-term options for the management of national health care systems. But this influence derives considerable sustenance from the existence of concrete institutional bases. In most industrialized societies a hierarchy of interest groups tends to reproduce the status system of the workplace in a wider arena provided by the State.

The nature of medical control over the delivery process and over the deployment of clinical knowledge is, as a number of contributions have suggested, changing and, perhaps, eroding. It remains the case that the creation of a managerial hierarchy capable of designing and delivering health care services, or, in the terms used by institutional economists, of 'appropriating the idiosyncratic information assets' (Williamson, 1985) of the medical professions, is, to say the least, problematic.

The solution contained in the analysis of Professor Enthoven (1985) was that of matching the market-oriented structures of closed occupational hierarchies with that of a regulated market place. In cultural terms this might equally as well be expressed in terms of matching the individualist ideology of professional organization based on the concept of 'job property' with the means of testing the value of this property. In the USA and France, the medical profession formed early alliances with university facilities in regulating the supply of educated labour as well as in the accreditation and monitoring of standards of service in hospitals and elsewhere (Jamous and Peloille, 1970). The creation of private health care insurance agencies has tended to distance the providers from direct regulation by the state, although both states appear to have more overt regulatory procedures than are present in the 'highway code' approach adopted in this country. In the UK the role of the state as both provider and regulator of delivery systems has been exercised at national level in close, if somewhat erratic, collaboration with the Royal Colleges and through numerous elitist networks (Parry and Parry, 1976).

By grossly over-simplifying these complex relationships involved in the strategic management of health care, it is possible to illustrate the options available to decision makers along two significant dimensions. These are illustrated in Fig. 15.1 which is adapted from Elridge and Crombie's (1974) attempt to juxtapose the effects of *internal* competition between groups within organizations and *external* competition in inter-organizational relationships. Along the vertical axis is measured the concentration of power within the internal hierarchy. This may be either concentrated at the top in a well-defined elite group holding strategic control or diffused across a number of power bases at the operational levels of the organization.

If one follows the logic of contingency theory this power axis is likely to relate to one in which the technical knowledge of the system's workings is either predominantly held by a strategic elite as in a rational bureaucracy or, contrawise, is highly dependent on the operational expertise of those lower in the hierarchy as in a craft or professionally administered system. Perrow (1970), for example, sees hospitals as typically examples of devolved power or polyarchy.

The horizontal axis represents the degree of monopoly/competition presented by the environment of the organization. This in turn might

Figure 15.1 The nature of governance within given internal/external
organizational interfaces

Relations within the organization

Power (knowledge) concentrated at top of hierarchy

	Permanent elite	Circulating elites

Relations between
organizations   Public   Free
(variability)   monopoly   competition

	Factional polyarchy	Local oligarchy

Diffused power
(knowledge)

be expressed as contributing to the contingent element of variability or
strategic uncertainty facing the organization's managers.

The UK NHS might be seen as one in which a public monopoly had
given rise to a permanent elite of the (former) DHSS administrators
consulting with the respective professional elites at each of the geographi-
cally defined levels of decision-making, RHA and DHA. Their continuation in office has been assured by what Michels (1914, 1962 edition) has
defined as the 'iron law of oligarchy'. Within communally representative
organizations such as the NHS, elected representatives are likely to be
transient and therefore highly dependent on permanent civil servants for
their knowledge of how the system works and of the normative constraints for decision making. Meanwhile the existence of public monopoly
had created an arena within which professional experts could bid for funds
to support their specialization with no price constraints. In fact, medical
consultants have had direct access to the same political constituency as that
to which transient political representatives had also to appeal for support,
i.e. the local community. Given the lack of clear budgetary feedback from
their actions there was every incentive for clinical experts to maximize
their bids for local funds at the expense of the whole. (Anyone with recent
experience in higher education will recognize similar propensities.) Given
also the lack of expertise or willingness to set strategic priorities among
the permanent administrative elite in the context of such a politically

sensitive arena, it was natural that the direction of innovation should be determined as the outcome of a factional struggle at the operational level of the organization. (Again a not unknown phenomenon in higher education!)

The 1990 Act has endorsed the earlier pressure towards the appointment of a circulating elite of professional management recommended in the first Griffiths Report by changing the basis of representation on 'boards of directors' at all levels of the NHS. Instead of being comprised of elected or nominated representatives from elected authorities together with career civil servants, they are to more closely resemble an executive board of a private company, employed on a short-term contract and adjudged in terms of the operational success of the firm.

At the local level the survival of the strategic operational unit, be it a hospital or general practice, will depend upon the collaboration of general managers (formerly administrators) and the senior professionals. In other words the internal hierarchy of the operational unit is to gain ascendancy both in day-to-day operations and in the long-term allocation of resources, over broader loyalties to occupational careers and to professional peers in the 'invisible college'. The oligarchy might more closely resemble that of the US hospital in which the medical team works alongside the senior administrator and fund-raiser. Though this is not a model that is presently being followed it is apparent that the latter function is intended both to enhance the power of the unit general manager and to bring about a new *localized* ordering of agreed priorities in the selection of capital projects and in external appeals to the public constituency for their support.

How far can health care be managed?

Clearly, the 'internal market' system introduced on 1 April 1991 has not moved the NHS far towards freeing competition between provider units. Indeed, even in the strategic regulation of hospital-trusts and budget-holding practices, Area and Regional Boards continue to exercise considerable authority. Nor are the reforms intended to be purely structural. Changes in the role and education of health service managers have been attempted with a view to bringing about a change in their perceptual horizons.

As Cox has pointed out earlier (Chapter 2), the concept of 'managerialism' can be treated as little more than the basis for an ideology by which to justify more central control over the operations of the services. Nevertheless like any professional claim to power, managers have to back their bid for status by the assembly of a coherent body of knowledge and range of operational techniques. General management does not have to provide for a detailed operational knowledge of the product or process being delivered. The scepticism expressed by the RCN in their mid-1980s advertising campaign was reported earlier by Cox in the phrase 'an aging accountant with the clip-board does not know his coccyx from his humerus'. Equally it might be said that Arnold Weinstock's knowledge of the solid-state physics practised by GEC might be taken as fairly insubstantial in the judgement of any junior physicist in that company's employ. On the other hand, his strategic knowledge of the organization's operations must go beyond that based on a few, supposedly, 'key' indicators.

As Coombes and Cooper have pointed out (Chapter 9) management that stops short at the mere application of narrow accountancy criteria to the production of clinical services (or indeed to the operations of GEC for that matter) would be ultimately destructive to the provision of those services. Furthermore, the pioneering management information systems imported from the USA show little recognition of cost differences between the diversity of services offered by the average district general hospital in the UK and have not penetrated apparently 'imponderable' aspects of diagnostic and treatment procedures (Ellwood, 1990). We might therefore pause to consider against this evident lack of 'progress' in the US application of scientific management to health care delivery whether the UK Government are once more attempting to follow the wrong exemplar? Is such a detailed evaluation of medical output in the NHS – and therefore the detailed monitoring of its activities – either feasible or necessary?

The answer hinted at by Coombes and Cooper, and attempted on trial sites in the 1980s, is that of the co-optation of clinicians and general practitioners into the management of their own operations. This may be seen as a process that has begun in the near locality of the clinical department or general practice but which may well ascend progressively through the evolution of professional career ladders into strategic management. As these authors have already suggested there is a most profound uncertainty surrounding the eventual merger of medical and managerial hierarchies within the NHS. This must include the adjustment of values and belief systems that have grown up over more than a century of increasingly complex bureaucracy within health care administration.

These tensions are expressed differently in different situations and at various levels of the care delivery system. Mok (1987) has expressed his analysis of these forces in a two-dimensional illustration. In Fig. 15.2, the level of autonomy exercised in the workplace is measured in terms of the amount of control felt by the service provider over the conceptual basis for carrying out a particular task within its overall context. At the opposite pole the operative control is limited to the application of a particular skill or technique within the workplace. These are performed in relation to certain procedures. Procedures may be either technical and having to do with the design of one's product or they may be regulatory or having to do with the way one relates to the total organization.

Recent studies by psychologists tend to support the importance of recognizing these separate dimensions of work autonomy and control in the design of organizations (Breaugh, 1989). What is described as *task*

Figure 15.2 Dimensions of occupational autonomy (Mok, 1987)

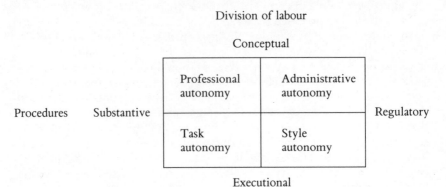

Division of labour

Conceptual

Professional autonomy	Administrative autonomy
Task autonomy	Style autonomy

Procedures   Substantive   Regulatory

Executional

autonomy is to be found in many posts for technically qualified staff in the NHS. Evidently those working in primary care tend to enjoy more autonomy in carrying out their tasks as a result of physical remoteness from administrative control. Even so, almost all concerned with the provision of a direct service, including all ward staff, exercise a large measure of control over their *style* of transacting with clients. Case studies such as that of Grieco demonstrate (Chapter 14) the vocation that many qualified nurses feel for offering direct patient care. What has to be questioned is the extent of their desire to exercise administrative autonomy beyond the level of their task situation. Perhaps equally, if not more, questionable is the actual nature of the autonomy afforded to, say, devolved budget holders under the new arrangements. In practice the boundaries to their influence over resource allocation have, by virtue of this 'devolution of power,' become strictly and overtly prescribed by the devolvers higher in the managerial hierarchy.

Moreover it implies the doctors' acceptance of the evaluation of the *outputs* from clinical procedures by reference to performance standards derived from totally alien disciplines, most importantly those of welfare and managerial economics. While these may have no direct effects on the *inputs* of medical knowledge and skills called upon in diagnosing and treating patients, they may ultimately create pressures for particular lines of activity to be pursued to the detriment of less measurable paths or those offering less immediate success.

Above all they remove such strategic judgements outside of the limited domain of the professionally qualified into one in which all who accept the validity of such measures can claim equal right to make judgement. By endorsing the basis for measurement of its members' performance, in this way the professional association thereby loses one of the most important instruments of control over those members.

Towards an integration of logics

In fact, a range of social and technical pressures is building up that are likely to breach the boundary between professional and managerial roles. Technical change within the task environment is part of the expected nature of medicine. However, the growing degree of medical specialization within the professional division of labour has brought increasing complexity to clinical management. When combined with a growing inadequacy in the supply of educated labour, a decline that will accelerate over the first part of the 1990s because of demographic trends, the devolution of tasks to less-qualified staff appears inevitable. Hence the long struggle for recognition among paramedicals, such as pharmacists and nurse practitioners described earlier in the volume, is likely to meet with increasingly positive recognition. The greater articulation of the relative costs of clinical procedures will bring a new perspective on situations in which the brief appearance of a doctor to 'rubber-stamp' treatment procedures has lost all but a ritualistic significance. Within general practice the increased role of GPs in health maintenance programmes has caused many to devolve such public educational roles to practice nurses in the manner described by Bryden (Chapter 5).

When taken together with their increased role in the coordination of community nursing and liaising with Local Authorities in other aspects of community care, the need of the GP for managerial expertise becomes more and more apparent. Although a separate role for the business manager has emerged, accompanied by the inevitable entourage of ritually qualifying associations, there is little evidence of the doctor wishing to relinquish strategic control over either the management of general practice or the clinical unit. This being so, his or her ability to render a direct service to the client may be increasingly encroached upon by the need to orchestrate and conduct the provision of a collective service given by specialist clinical and paramedical staff. Much the same pattern can be observed within the clinical departments of hospitals where members of the clinical team have often a well institutionalized division of labour in the performance of administrative tasks.

Of possibly even greater consequence is the emergence of different patterns of nursing. In extended periods of observation on wards in a major teaching hospital and a district general hospital in the mid-1980s, the author discovered that the normal, though officially unrecognized, pattern was often for qualified nurses to be acting as supervisor over a ward staff complement of nursing auxiliaries, sometimes on night shifts being responsible for up to three wards at a time. With the launch of the service-wide programme of upgrading formal nurse training and education in the latter part of the 1980s, more opportunities became available for experienced auxiliaries to advance their careers. Against this the demands of off-ward training became such as to intensify the need for unqualified substitutes over that period.

There seems little doubt that the articulation of nursing costs provided by the many new management information systems (MIS) now on offer have reinforced administrative pressures for the employment of unqualified nursing auxiliaries. Perhaps of even greater consequence is the claim that most such MIS systems make in regard to the flexible deployment of available nursing staff in accordance to a defined centralized hospital requirement. The logics of such systems run contrary to the prevailing ethos of local and professional task specialization and loyalties associated with attachment of individual nurses to particular teams or consultancy 'firms' and, more importantly, to the growing specialization in postgraduate training.

What may be seen as occurring is a growing polarization of the NHS work-force. Those service providers who hold specialized knowledge can be seen to exercise an increasingly managerial role in the coordination of lowly skilled direct service providers (i.e. nursing auxiliaries, porters etc.) as well as intervening periodically in a diagnostic or treating role. As such they may be increasingly isolated from the patient and more occupied with resource allocation. At present, considerable scope exists for choice in professional vocation. Paradoxically it could well be the case that the historical success of the professional institutions in appropriating managerial knowledge to their members could ensure the continuation of that choice.

Coda

Although at first resisted as threatening to established personal expectations and norms of practice, the creation of the internal market may find increased support from among those whose professional calling contains a fine balance of instrumentalism and moral commitment. Administrative changes, which over the last 20 years have appeared to threaten the task and style autonomy of professional workers may gain new significance as they become transformed into conceptual tools with which to advance their status and market position through engagement and identity with new management roles.

On the other hand, for the officers of the Royal Colleges and other professional associations the costs involved in the defence of their members' traditional privileges whilst attempting to retain the personal commitment of those members could be very great. Bolstered by the implicit, as well as formal, recognition of their representative role at all levels of the old NHS structure they may find the new conditions sap their managerial capabilities as much, if not more, than did the last decade of change within NHS administration. The willingness of their individual members to accept change may well run ahead of the ability of their associations to channel and orchestrate it in the manner that they have succeeded in doing for nearly two centuries. This could result in a build-up of institutional conflict as a background to workplace change.

This last chapter has attempted to place the attempts to achieve the organizational reform of the NHS which have occurred over the past decade into perspective. A brief comparison of the polar strategies adopted by three different industrialized countries in adjusting to the crises in welfare provision has been made. The organization of health care delivery around the opposite poles of market and hierarchy were described as leading to a remarkable congruence in some specific outcomes over recent years. In all cases the managerial agents had failed to contain the costs of service provision and technological development. The mode of reform adopted by the Thatcher administration has been presented in this analysis as the use of a regulatory framework within which limited market pressures are to be used to create a more proactive managerial frame. By the same token it has been suggested that a greater congruence in commitment and occupational stance may occur between professional and administrative perspectives. This is not to offer any commentary on its effect on the expression of community or client needs or upon the values represented in pre-existing institutions. As a mode of control its efficiency will ultimately have to be judged by the consumer, or by the client acting as citizen in the political arena.

References

Breaugh, J.A. (1989) The work autonomy scales: additional validity evidence. *Human Relations*, **42**(11), 1033–56.

Child, J. and Loveridge, R. (1990) *Information Technology in European Services: Towards a Microelectronic Future*. Oxford: Basil Blackwell.

Ellwood, S. (1990) Competition in health care. *Management Accounting*, April, 24–8.

Elridge, J.E.T. and Crombie, A.D. (1974) *A Sociology of Organizations*. London: Allen & Unwin.

Enthoven, A. (1985) *Reflections on the Management of the National Health Service*. London: Nuffield Provincial Hospitals Trust.

Jamous, H. and Peloille, B. (1970) Changes in the French university-hospital system. In: *Professions and Professionalism*, Jackson, J.A. (ed.). Cambridge: Cambridge University Press.

Kuttner, R. (1991) Health care: why corporate America is paralyzed. *Business Week*, 8 April, 8.

Michels, R. (1914, 1962 edn) *Political Parties – A Sociological Study of the Oligarchical Tendencies of Modern Democracy*. London: Collier.

Mok, A.L. (1987) Autonomy and professional work. In: *Technology as the Two-edged Sword. Proceedings of the European Group on Organisational Studies Colloquium*. Free University of Antwerp, July.

Parry, N. and Parry, J. (1976) *The Rise of the Medical Profession*. London: Croom Helm.

Perrow, C. (1970) *Organizational Analysis: a Sociological View*. London: Tavistock.

Pollitt, C., Hams, S., Hunt, D. and Marnoch, G. (1988) The reluctant manager: clinicians and budgets in the NHS. *Financial Accountability and Management*, **4** (III), pp. 213–33.

Williamson, O.E. (1985) *The Economic Institutions of Capitalism*. New York: Free Press.

Index